THE HUMAN NAIL
Ailments and Diseases
Symptoms, Causes, and Treatment

Pierre Mouchette

Life Knowledge Media USA
An Enviro | Life Knowledge Publication
a subsidiary of Real Property Experts LLC

THE HUMAN NAIL - Ailments and Diseases
Symptoms, Causes, and Treatment

Copyright © 2022 by Pierre Mouchette

All rights reserved. No part of this publication may be reproduced, distributed, or transmitted in any form or by any means, including photocopying, recording, or other electronic or mechanical methods, without the prior written permission of the publisher, except in the case of brief quotations embodied in critical reviews and specific other noncommercial uses permitted by copyright law.

ISBN 979-8834954156 (Paperback Book)

Independently Published

First Edition: June 2022
Life Knowledge Media USA
An Enviro | Life Knowledge Publication
Web Address: https://www.enviro-life-media.com
Contact: publications@rpe4u.com

Note: This publication comes in various formats, such as Paperbacks and Electronic Books (e-books). Some material in the paperback version of this book may not be included in e-books, and vice versa.

At Life Knowledge Media USA, we pride ourselves on every publication's quality, research, and transparency. All content is thoroughly researched.

THE HUMAN NAIL - Ailments and Diseases
Symptoms, Causes, and Treatment

DISCLAIMER

This Life Knowledge Media USA publication provides information about the subject matter covered. The author and publisher of this content are not acting as licensed professionals to present the covered material. The information and statements made are for educational purposes and are not intended to replace a one-on-one relationship with a qualified attorney, accountant, tax professional, or other licensed professionals. You are solely responsible for the use of any content. You hold Real Property Experts LLC, its subsidiaries, and members harmless in any event or claim, demand, or damage, including reasonable attorneys' fees, asserted by any third party, or arising out of your use of, or conduct on, publications and products.

Life Knowledge Media USA writers provide applicable content and break down complex topics so they are easier to understand. Information given may not apply to your specific situation, and products or services recommended may not be a good fit for your application. While Life Knowledge Media USA strives to provide accurate, up-to-date content, we cannot guarantee the accuracy and completeness of the information supplied. By using this content, you understand that all material is an expression of opinion and not professional advice.

THE HUMAN NAIL - Ailments and Diseases
Symptoms, Causes, and Treatment

PREFACE

Dystrophic nails are fingernails or toenails which are deformed, thickened, or discolored. There are many reasons for nail dystrophy, ranging from toenail fungus (onychomycosis) to skin conditions (psoriasis).

Some common problems of nail dystrophy include:

- Fingernails which are cracked, split, flaky, peeling, crumbly, and shed

- Nails that are misshapen or curved in an unusual way

- Nails that are thicker than usual or that are yellow, white, or brown in color

- Nails that are painful when encountering other objects

- Nails that are pulling away from or coming off your skin

Self-consciousness about nails leads to withdrawal from public and social situations

Nail dystrophy is an unattractive and profoundly concerning issue. It can be challenging to manage, but one of the best ways is to use early intervention. The earlier you work dealing with nail dystrophy, the better the outcome for any affected nails as they re-grow and recover.

If you have nail dystrophy and it is severe enough, it may require a prescription treatment to keep it under control. Learn more about the conditions and available treatments by reading this book. You will become aware of the various problems associated with human nails and how to protect and care for your nails.

For comments on this publication, please write to us at publications@rpe4u.com.

THE HUMAN NAIL - Ailments and Diseases
Symptoms, Causes, and Treatment

Contents

Section 1 **FINGERNAILS and TOENAILS** .... - 7 -
    Human Fingernails and Toenails .... - 8 -
    Caring For Your Nails .... - 13 -
    Nail Growth .... - 16 -
    Nail Biting .... - 19 -
    Fingernail and Toenail Problems .... - 21 -
    Nail Ailment vs. Nail Disease .... - 28 -

Section 2 **VITAMIN DEFICIENCIES and YOUR NAILS** - 29 -
    Vitamin Deficiencies Affect Your Nails .... - 30 -

Section 3 **NAIL AILMENTS and DISEASES** .... - 32 -
    Loose Nails .... - 34 -
    Black Toenails .... - 37 -
    Brittle Nails .... - 40 -
    Clubbing (curved nails) .... - 42 -
    Cracked, Split, Brittle Nails .... - 45 -
    Ingrown Toenails .... - 49 -
    Koilonychia (spoon-shaped nails) .... - 54 -
    Nail Fungus .... - 56 -
    Nail-Patella Syndrome .... - 59 -
    Nail Pitting .... - 60 -
    Nail Psoriasis .... - 62 -
    Onychoschizia (nail ridges) .... - 65 -
    Onychogryphosis (ram's horn nails) .... - 70 -
    Onycholysis (loose nails) .... - 74 -
    Onychomycosis (thick toenails) .... - 78 -

THE HUMAN NAIL - Ailments and Diseases
Symptoms, Causes, and Treatment

Onychophosis (callus build-up) ....- 82 -
Onychoschizia (split nails) ....- 84 -
Paronychia (nail/skin infections) ....- 88 -
Stubbed Toe ....- 91 -
Subungual Hematoma ....- 92 -
Turf Toe ....- 95 -
Yellow Toenails ....- 98 -

Section 4   **HOME REMEDIES** ....- 101 -
     Ingrown Toenail ....- 102 -
     Nail Dystrophy ....- 103 -
     Nail Fungus (onychomycosis) ....- 104 -
     Nail Splitting, Brittle, Soft (onychoschizia) ....- 107 -
     Paronychia (nail/skin infections) ....- 108 -
     Stubbed Toe ....- 109 -

Section 5   **NAIL POLISH and TOXIC CHEMICALS** ......- 110 -
     Being Trendy ....- 111 -
     Nail Polish and Toxins ....- 112 -

APPENDIX A ....- 115 -
     Must-Know Words and Phrases ....- 116 -
     So That You Know ....- 118 -

THE HUMAN NAIL - Ailments and Diseases
Symptoms, Causes, and Treatment

Section 1
FINGERNAILS and TOENAILS

THE HUMAN NAIL - Ailments and Diseases
Symptoms, Causes, and Treatment

Human Fingernails and Toenails

In most primates, a nail is a claw-like plate at the tip of the fingers and toes. Human nails correspond to the claws found in other animals. Fingernails and toenails consist of a tough protective protein called alpha-keratin that also occurs in the skin and hair.

The Fingers
A hand is a prehensile, multi-fingered appendage located at the end of the forearm or forelimb of humans. Five digits (fingers) are attached to each hand, with a nail fixed to the ends.

There are two thumbs, each located on one of the sides of the hand parallel with the arm. A reliable method of identifying human hands is the presence of opposable thumbs. Opposable thumbs are identified by the ability to be brought opposite to the fingers, a muscle action known as opposition.

All four fingers can be folded over the palm, allowing for grasping objects. Each finger, starting with the one closest to the thumb, has a colloquial name to distinguish it from the others:

- Index finger (pointer finger/forefinger), or 2nd digit
- The middle finger (long finger) or 3rd digit
- Ring finger or 4th digit
- Little finger (pinky finger/small finger/baby finger), or 5th digit

The Toes
The toe refers to a part of the human foot, with five toes present on each foot. The hallux is the first toe of the foot, also called the big toe, because its appearance is more prominent than the other toes of the foot. This big toe is also known as the thumb

toe or leg thumb. Each toe, starting with the one closest to the hallux, has a colloquial name to distinguish it from the others:

- The index/pointer toe (the second toe)
- The middle toe (the long toe)
- The ring toe (the fourth toe)
- The outermost/pinky toe (the small toe)

Attached to the end of all five toes is a toenail.

Nails Provide Several Vital Purposes
They help humans to function. They are flat versions of claws that help humans dig, climb, scratch, grab, and more.

Nails guard against injuries by serving as a protective plate, helping to prevent the fingers from cuts and scrapes during daily activities.

In addition, the nails:

- **Enhance sensations** - the fingers have nerve endings that allow the mind to process the information it receives every time something is touched. Nails function as a counterforce, providing even more sensory input after someone feels something.

- The nails protect the tip of the fingers and toes from trauma and help a person grab and hold small objects as a unit.

Nail Growth
Human nails are constantly growing, but their growth rate slows down due to poor blood circulation and aging. Production of new nail cells is constant, with new cells keratinizing and forcing the old cells toward the nail surface.

THE HUMAN NAIL - Ailments and Diseases
Symptoms, Causes, and Treatment

The nail cell matrix is continuously dividing by mitosis, with the plate growing continually throughout one's life. It can take six months for a fingernail to grow from the root to the free edge, and toenails grow much more slowly from 12 to 18 months.

Nail Structure

The nail structure comprises several components: root, nail bed, nail plate, eponychium, paronychium, and hyponychium. Each has a specific function, and if a component of the nail structure is disrupted, the nail can look abnormal.

- **Nail root** - the nail root (germinal matrix) appears as a white crescent, known as the **lunula.** The root portion lies below the skin, underneath the nail, and extends into the finger. The root produces most of the nail and the nail bed volume.

- **Nail bed** - the nail bed (sterile matrix) ranges from the edge of the nail root (lunula) to the **hyponychium.** Nail beds contain blood vessels, nerves, and **melanocytes** that produce **melanin.** As the nail root grows, the nail streams down along the nail bed and adds material to the underside of the nail, making it thicker. As the nail grows appropriately, the nail bed is smooth. But if the nail does not grow properly, the nail may split or develop ridges that are not cosmetically attractive.

- **Nail plate** - or the **fingernail,** is made up of translucent **keratin.** The pinkish appearance comes from the blood vessels beneath the plate. The bottom sides of the nail plate have grooves that run along the length of the nail, helping to anchor it to the nail bed.

- **Eponychium** - more commonly known as the **cuticle,** is situated between the skin of the finger and the nail plate. It fuses these structures and provides a waterproof barrier.

- **Paronychium** - is the skin that overlaps onto the sides of the nail plate, also known as the **paronychial edge.** The paronychium is the location of hangnails, ingrown nails, and **paronychia,** a skin infection.

- **Hyponychium** - is the area between the free edge of the nail plate and the fingertip's skin. It provides a waterproof barrier.

Things To Be Aware Of

Nails can reveal certain aspects of a person's health. The nail might develop white spots if a nail bed is injured, although these spots diminish over time. Some other indications can be more serious. For example, one symptom of psoriasis's inflammatory skin condition is separating the nail plate from the bed. A response to certain medications can also cause this same symptom.

People with diabetes should be especially cautious of nail injuries or infections in the nail bed. A doctor's examination should be scheduled to confirm a diagnosis and then continue with treatment as with any medical condition. Indications of an infection include redness, swelling, pressure, and a hot or burning feeling in or around the nail.

While not all nail bed problems are avoidable, specific steps can help protect them from damage and infection. Habits such as nail-biting and chewing should be avoided, as they can directly damage the nail bed and allow microbes to enter the nail. Nail polish remover must be used sparingly, as it tends to dry out the nail, leading to the splitting of the nail and the introduction of bacteria.

THE HUMAN NAIL - Ailments and Diseases
Symptoms, Causes, and Treatment

Using a nail hardener is an excellent way to help build up the strength of the entire nail. It will protect the bed as well. Healthy nail beds help keep the whole nail intact and smooth, which results in nice-looking nails with improved sensation and dexterity in the fingers.

Caring For Your Nails

How To Clip Your Nails

Fingernails should be clipped square with round edges, while toenails need to be cut straight across slightly above the tip of the toes. File nails with an emery board engaged in one direction from side to center. Only buff your nails in the direction of nail growth. Going in the other direction can lead to splitting. Nails need to be cleaned weekly with soap and a nail brush or a soft bristle toothbrush.

What To and Not To Do To Care For Your Nails?

Some Do's for nail care are:

- Apply moisturizer daily at night on the nail and proximal nail fold to keep them shiny.

- Buy shoes that have enough space for toe movements.

- Clean nails with nail tools.

- Remove all nail polish at least fortnightly and apply moisturizer.

- Wear gloves when doing household work, especially if your nails are brittle.

Some DO NOTs for nail care are:

- Do not grow your fingernails too long because that increases the chances of separating the nail plate from the nail bed.

THE HUMAN NAIL - Ailments and Diseases
Symptoms, Causes, and Treatment

- Do not overuse nail polish remover because the acetone or alcohol content can weaken and dry the nails.

- Do not pull or tear at hanging nails. Always cut your nails, leaving the cuticle intact.

- Do not immerse your nails in water or detergent water for too long.

- Do not use fingernails as a tool.

Maintain a Healthy Diet
Your diet is essential to healthy skin and nails.

- **Balanced Diet** - maintain a balanced and nutritious diet that includes (fruits, vegetables, whole grains), proteins, iron, and vitamins (especially Biotin) are excellent for nail health. Biotin may be found in eggs, milk, broccoli, cauliflower, bananas, lentils, fish, soybeans, cereals, and whole grains. Omega-3 fatty acids are essential for helping with ridges.

- **Healthy Foods** - avoid nutrient-poor processed and prepackaged junk foods. If you find yourself craving sugars or junk food, buy fresher or healthier ingredients to make it yourself at home.

- **Nutritional Supplements** - consume B12, zinc, and iron supplements associated with providing nutrition for deficiencies that cause fingernail problems.

- **Water Intake** - be sure to drink plenty of water each day. It will improve your overall health by supporting your body's organs and helping with waste elimination.

THE HUMAN NAIL - Ailments and Diseases
Symptoms, Causes, and Treatment

Take Care of Your Nails:

- **Manicure** - filing or buffing your fingernails gently with an emery board can help smooth out fingernail ridges. Be careful not to buff them harshly.

- **Cleaning and Moisturizing** - keep your nails clean to avoid fungus growth and moisturize your hands and cuticles. Consider using naturally rich oils like avocado oil, Jojoba oil, or shea butter. Select an item that will stay on your skin for a time. Moisturize nails and skin following water exposure and frequently throughout the day. Apply hydrating lotions or creams when your nails are dry and before bed.

- **Treating Injuries** - a nail injury such as closing the door on a finger or breaking the nail off the nail bed can cause nail ridges if you do not take care of the nail as it grows back. Trauma causes direct damage to the nail bed that requires treatment for healthy nail recovery.

- **Wearing Gloves** - if you are doing work around the house and are engaging detergents and other cleaning supplies, wear gloves so that your nails do not contact these products.

Note: well-maintained nails are less likely to have rough edges that snag on clothing or items. These snags can lead to splitting.

Nail Growth

Why Your Nails Are Not Growing

If your nails will not grow or have stopped growing, you might lack specific vitamins, proteins, and minerals in your diet, or it could be that you do not moisturize them well enough. The following are some reasons why your fingernails or toenails are not growing as expected:

- **You do not moisturize them enough** - moisturizing your nails is one of the most reliable methods of helping your nails to grow out well. To moisten means to apply ointment or cream to the nails and the skin surrounding the nail (cuticle).
  - The cuticle, when moisturized, helps protect the nails from intruding bacteria and creates an enabling environment for nail growth. All creams do not serve this purpose, and for this reason, you should use a cream rich in fats or lipids. These creams must be applied daily on the nails and cuticles for effective results, preferably three times a day.

- **You do not exercise enough** - if your nails suddenly stopped growing, then it could be that you do not make time to exercise. **'Regular exercise helps nails grow.'**
  - During a workout, the rate at which blood flows to the nail matrix increases, and when it happens, there is an increase in the growth of the fingernails and toenails.

- **You bite your nails** - constantly picking at your nails might be why your nails are not growing. When you bite the nails, you subject them to trauma, leading to underlying health challenges such as **onychomycosis,** a severe fungal infection that often slows nail growth.

THE HUMAN NAIL - Ailments and Diseases
Symptoms, Causes, and Treatment

- **You use your nails as tools** - although long nails can serve as a handy tool without having any, this act can cause lots of damage to the nails. Sometimes, the nail may lift away from the nail bed, stopping nail growth.

- **You lack a crucial nutrient in your diet** - this is another factor to consider when nails are not growing as expected or have suddenly stopped growing. Our diets play a significant role in nail growth. If your nails are continually splitting or they are brittle, it could be that you lack protein, iron, or zinc in your diet. Incorporating food such as broccoli, spinach, vegetables, whole grains, meat, eggs, or beans can help nails grow well.

- **Underlying health challenges** - underlying health conditions like kidney, psoriasis, thyroid, or liver disease can invariably be why your nails have stopped growing. So, if you are experiencing a pause in nail growth, it is wise to check your overall health condition with your doctor to know the cause.

- **You use nail polish too often** - if you want to see a leap in nail growth, you must stop or limit how you go about using nail polish. Nail polish contains active chemicals that can make your nails brittle and break. Additionally, acetone polish remover is another thing that inhibits nail growth.

- **Your medication might be the cause** - intake of some medications like chemotherapy could be what is interfering with your nail growth. Most often, the side effects of medications are the primary cause of significant nail growth problems. So, if you are experiencing no growth in your nails, visit your doctor to advise you on what to do.

THE HUMAN NAIL - Ailments and Diseases
Symptoms, Causes, and Treatment

Recommendations For Slow Growing Nails

- **Moisturize more** - when moisturizing, be sure to accompany it with a massage, helping blood flow to the nail matrix.

- **Do not cut your cuticle** - the cuticle plays a vital role in nail growth. However, the cuticle should not be cut or trimmed. If you feel it is too long, the best way is to push them back. Before moving them back using a cuticle pusher, be sure they are well moisturized to avoid tearing them apart. Torn cuticles can create an enabling environment for bacterial or fungal infections.

- **Avoid using harsh chemicals** - nail polishes, detergents, and hand sanitizers all contain chemicals capable of rendering nails brittle. If you do work that involves exposing the hands to chemicals, wear rubber gloves. For nail polishes, try to limit usage or go for chemical-free ones.

- **Eat healthily** - try to eat foods rich in the six food classes. Nails need a balanced diet to grow well. Incorporate foods rich in vitamins, calcium, minerals, and proteins into your diet. These foods help to strengthen the nails and improve nail growth.

Nail Biting

Although nail-biting is a widespread problem, it can be triggered by behaviors that range from stress to anxiety. While the behavior may seem simple to stop, many individuals who have attempted to break the habit have not succeeded. Instead, they experience unsightly nails, damage to the skin, and soreness surrounding the nail bed.

What Causes Nail-Biting?
Nail-biting (onychophagia) is also known as pathological grooming. It can be a behavior of obsessive-compulsive disorders (OCDs). Nail-biting can begin through stress, anxiety, boredom, and mental health disorders.

- **Stress and Anxiety** - may be triggered by events. Unlike physical reactions, such as a pounding heart or hyperventilating, which can result in a fight-or-flight response, nail-biting releases stress and anxiety because it feels good.

- **Boredom and frustration** - can also trigger the need to do something instead of nothing. A perfectionist personality can bring on this type of behavior.

- **Mental Health Disorders** - are body-focused repetitive behavior disorders listed under obsessive-compulsive disorder.

Behaviors of these types can disrupt one's day-to-day activities and personal interactions. Not acting out on compulsive behavior causes further distress rather than relief. In the case of compulsive nail-biting, it feels good and releases stress.

Other disorders that the nail biter may have include:

- Attention deficit hyperactivity disorder (ADHD)
- Genetics
- Oppositional defiant disorder (when an individual is rebellious and disobedient towards people of authority)
- Separation anxiety disorder
- Tourette's syndrome

Side Effects and Risks of Nail Biting

Nail-biting has many physical and psychological side effects, which include:

- Damaging cuticle and surrounding skin; redness and soreness
- Dental issues
- Long-term, habitual nail-biting can disrupt natural nail growth and cause deformed nails.
- Possible bacterial infection in the nail beds and mouth
- Problems with relationships
- Psychological issues with self-esteem, shame, depression

When To See Your Doctor

An infrequent nibble on your nails might not require visiting a doctor, but if the nail beds are infected and have spread to your mouth, you need treatment with antibiotics.

How to Stop Nail Biting

To get out of the nail-biting habit or treat long-term nail-biting that results from psychological disorders, **cognitive behavioral therapy (CBT)** may help.

THE HUMAN NAIL - Ailments and Diseases
Symptoms, Causes, and Treatment

Fingernail and Toenail Problems

Where You Can Get Help
Nails support and protect the sensitive tips of our fingers and toes. Fingernails also help us pick up items, scratch an itch or untangle a knot. Fingernails grow three times quicker than toenails.

Nail problems have an impact on people of all ages. Diet is not responsible for abnormal nail changes unless the individual suffers from severe malnutrition. Some nail conditions will require professional treatment from either a **podiatrist** or a **dermatologist,** but others will respond to simple self-help techniques and minor lifestyle changes. When in doubt about a condition, seek your **primary doctor's** help.

Toenail problems can impact people of all ages but tend to be more common in older adults. Reasons for fingernail problems might involve **injury, infection,** and **skin diseases** such as **eczema** and **psoriasis.** Toenail issues include **trauma, ill-fitting shoes, poor circulation, poor nerve supply,** and **infection.** A podiatrist can successfully treat toenail problems.

Nail Structure
Nails are made from **keratin,** the same protein as skin and hair use. Nails grow from the cells that multiply within the base of the nail, then layer on top of each other and harden. The process is called keratinization.

Strength, thickness, and the growth rate of nails are traits inherited from our parents. The structure of the nail includes:

- **Nail matrix** - this is where nail growth is taking place, under the skin behind the nail

THE HUMAN NAIL - Ailments and Diseases
Symptoms, Causes, and Treatment

- **Nail plate** - visible portion of a nail

- **Nail bed** - the nail plate rests on top of the nail bed. The nail plate looks pink due to the blood-rich capillaries in the nail bed

- **Lunula** - the crescent-moon shape located at the base of the nail plate

- **Nail folds** - the skin grooves that keep the nail plate in place

- **Cuticle** - the thin tissue over the base of the nail plate

Nail Disorders
Many conditions can affect nails, with different causes and treatments.

Nail Discoloration
A healthy nail plate is pink, and the nail looks white as it grows off the nail bed. Causes of discolored nails typically include:

- Certain infections
- Hair-coloring agents
- Injury to the nail bed
- Lifted nail plate
- Melanoma
- Nail polish
- Nicotine from cigarette smoking
- Some medications, including antibiotics, anti-malarial drugs, and some medicines used in chemotherapy

THE HUMAN NAIL - Ailments and Diseases
Symptoms, Causes, and Treatment

Nail color change - a disease inside your body can cause your nails to change color. Specific color changes can be a warning sign of a particular disease.

Color	Disease or other health problem
Blue half-moons	It could be a sign of poisoning
Blue nails	Not enough oxygen in your bloodstream
Dusky red half-moons	It could be lupus, heart disease, alopecia areata, arthritis, dermatomyositis
Half pink, half white nails	Kidney disease
Pale nails	Anemia
White nails	Liver disease, diabetes
Yellow nails	Lung disease, nail infection

When the nail plate lifts off the nail bed, it appears white. Common reasons include:

- Harsh removal of artificial nails
- Nail polishes that contain hardening chemicals like formalin
- Overenthusiastic cleaning under the nails
- Psoriasis
- Thickened nails
- Tinea (a fungal infection)

Such conditions affect the toenails more than the fingernails.

THE HUMAN NAIL - Ailments and Diseases
Symptoms, Causes, and Treatment

Older people are at greater risk. Causes include:

- Altered gait (walking) pattern
- Arthritis in the toes
- Fungal infection
- Ill-fitting shoes
- Injury
- Neglect
- Poor circulation
- Psoriasis
- Ridged nails

Ridges that run the length or width of the nail plate may have several causes, including:

- Age-related changes
- Eczema
- Fever or illness
- Lichen planus infection
- Overzealous attention to the cuticles
- Peripheral vascular disease
- Rheumatoid arthritis
- Trauma to the nail matrix

Bacterial Infection Of The Nail

Staphylococcus aureus bacterium is a common cause of bacterial infections of the nail. Typically, the condition first takes hold in the skin fold at the base of the nail (proximal nail fold). Untreated infections can get worse, leading to inflammation and pus. This bacterium is often associated with candida infection, particularly when it becomes chronic.

Activities that predispose someone to a bacterial nail infection include:

- Eczema around the fingernails

- Having constantly wet hands
- Overzealous attention to the cuticles
- Severe nail-biting, which can expose underlying tissues to infection

Congenital Disorders Of Nails

Certain nail conditions are congenital (present at birth). It includes nail-patella syndrome, in which the nails are ill-formed or lacking.

Deformed or Brittle Nails

Violent toe-stubbing, dropping a heavy object on the toe, or other trauma can injure the nail bed causing the nail to grow in a deformed manner. The nail may be thickened or ridged. Brittle and thickened nails can also be a normal aging process.

Deformed or brittle toenails will benefit from routine attention by a professional. **Cutting, shaping,** and **nail care** from a podiatrist will help improve the health of toenails, and the doctor can also diagnose and treat any nail problems.

Diseases And The Nails

Some diseases that can affect the shape, integrity, and color of the nails include:

- Heart disease
- Kidney disease
- Liver disease
- Lung disease
- Thyroid disease

THE HUMAN NAIL - Ailments and Diseases
Symptoms, Causes, and Treatment

Leukonychia (white spots) - are nonuniform white spots or lines on the nail. They are usually the result of minor trauma and are harmless in healthy individuals. Sometimes leukonychia is related to bad health or nutritional deficiency. Factors include infectious, metabolic, or systemic diseases and certain drugs.

Nail Tumors
Nails can be affected by tumors, including squamous cell carcinoma, usually caused by human papillomavirus (HPV) infection. Melanoma can also affect the nail.

Old Age And Nails
As our body ages, the growth rate of our fingernails and toenails tends to slow. The protein change in the nail plate makes nails brittle and prone to splitting. Discoloration and thickening are also common.

Splinter Hemorrhages Of The Nail
These are fine lines of blood moving along the nail bed. Causes may include injury, severe anemia, infective endocarditis (inflammation of the inner tissue of the heart), and certain diseases such as rheumatoid arthritis.

Swelling Of The Skin Alongside The Nail
The skin lying alongside the nail can become infected with bacteria, typically Staphylococcus aureus. This infection is called **paronychia**. Symptoms may include pain, redness, swelling around the cuticle, and a yellow-green secretion.

THE HUMAN NAIL - Ailments and Diseases
Symptoms, Causes, and Treatment

Diagnosis And Treatment Of Nail Problems

Abnormal changes in nails need to be investigated. See your doctor for treatment. If the cause of the nail problem is not apparent, your doctor will take nail clippings and scrapings from under the nail for laboratory analysis. Fingernail infections usually respond more quickly to treatment than toenail infections.

Depending upon the cause, treatment may include:

- Advice on appropriate nail care
- Antibiotics for bacterial infections
- Antifungal preparations
- Self-help strategies for healthy nails
- Treatment for any contributing skin disease

Methods to reduce the risk of nail problems include:

- Avoid harsh chemicals like strong soap and detergent
- Avoid or limit the handling of chemicals
- Be diligent in the use of nail polish
- Do not bite your nails
- Do not clean under your nails too often or too aggressively
- Moisturize hands frequently, especially after washing them
- Protect yourself from fungal infections, do not share towels, and dry yourself thoroughly after bathing (particularly between the toes).
- Remove artificial nails carefully using the instructions provided by the manufacturer
- Resist the temptation to bite or tear off hangnails, use nail clippers
- Treat any sign of eczema on the hands promptly
- Wear protective gloves for wet jobs such as washing the dishes
- Wear shoes that are well-fitting and have plenty of room for air movement

THE HUMAN NAIL - Ailments and Diseases
Symptoms, Causes, and Treatment

Nail Ailment vs. Nail Disease

Ailment and disease are a cause of harm to the body. Ailments and diseases can change normal functioning and lead to many problems in the body.

When looking at the two terms, an ailment is not that serious, whereas a disease is a significant situation. Most disorders (conditions) can be cured using simple over-the-counter OTC medications or home remedies. On the other hand, diseases cannot be treated using home remedies or simple medications.

If suffering from an ailment, there is no need to rush to the doctor. However, a doctor's advice is immediately needed when one has a disease. You should follow the doctor's direction and take medications per the prescription.

THE HUMAN NAIL - Ailments and Diseases
Symptoms, Causes, and Treatment

Section 2
VITAMIN DEFICIENCIES and YOUR NAILS

Vitamin Deficiencies Affect Your Nails

Iron Deficiency Effects On Nail Growth

Everyone needs iron to manufacture hemoglobin and myoglobin. These proteins are accountable for transporting oxygen to your tissues and muscles and your immune system's proper growth, development, and functioning. Iron deficiency is a widespread nutritional deficiency. An inadequate amount of iron in a diet will trigger poor iron absorption from the digestive tract or cause excessive bleeding, including heavy menstrual periods.

In addition to **fatigue, decreased body temperature,** and an **inflamed tongue,** iron deficiency also causes **brittle** and **splitting nails.** Foods containing iron include chicken liver, red meat, dark turkey meat, soybeans, and fortified cereals.

Zinc Deficiency

Although rare in developed countries, and with most cases due to an inherited condition, **acrodermatitis enteropathica** is caused by an inability to absorb zinc properly. Zinc is critical for growth and development and is necessary to produce over 100 different enzymes.

A zinc deficiency may be characterized by **delayed growth, frequent infections, slow-healing wounds, and brittle, splitting nails with white spots.** You could be at higher risk for a zinc deficiency if you are a vegetarian, have Crohn's disease, have other conditions causing malabsorption of nutrients, are pregnant, or are an alcoholic. Zinc may be found in oysters, beef, pork, yogurt, and beans.

Vitamin-A Deficiency

Vitamin-A is not one substance but a group of carotenoid compounds necessary to retain a **healthy immune system, vision, mucous membranes, and skin.** Vitamin-A levels have a direct impact on your levels of iron. Vitamin-A is required to transport iron from storage, so **inadequate vitamin-A levels create a functional deficiency.** As a result, you may also develop symptoms of **iron deficiency, including pale skin, fatigue,** and **brittle nails that split.**

Biotin For Nails

Although low levels of biotin will not cause brittle nails, supplementation with biotin seems to be effective in treating dry, brittle nails that split and peel. **Biotin, also called vitamin H, is one of the eight B vitamins.**

Biotin is recommended to remedy weak and splitting nails. There is, nevertheless, little evidence to support the claims. Obtain your healthcare provider's advice before taking biotin for brittle, splitting, and peeling nails.

Section 3
NAIL AILMENTS and DISEASES

THE HUMAN NAIL - Ailments and Diseases
Symptoms, Causes, and Treatment

Healthy nails are smooth and have consistent coloring. You might develop vertical ridges as you age, or your nails may be more brittle. It is usually harmless, and any spots due to injury should grow out.

Abnormalities such as spots, discoloration, and nail separation could result from injuries to fingers and hands, viral warts (periungual warts), infections (onychomycosis), and medications such as those used for chemotherapy.

Certain medical conditions might also change the appearance of the fingernails. However, these changes can be challenging to interpret. The fingernails' appearance is not sufficient to diagnose a specific illness. Your healthcare provider will use this information, other symptoms, and a physical exam to make a diagnosis. Always tell your doctor if you have questions about changes in your nails.

Nail Abnormalities
Some changes in the nails can be due to medical conditions needing attention, such as:

- A nail separating from the skin
- Any discoloration (dark streaks, white streaks, or changes in nail color)
- Bleeding around nails
- Changes in nail shape (curling or clubbing)
- Changes in nail thickness (thickening or thinning)
- Nails that become brittle or pit
- Pain around nails
- Swelling or redness around nails

The following pages will provide information on some of the more **common nail conditions, causes, symptoms, and how they are treated.**

Loose Nails

Fungal Infections
Nail fungal infections (**onycholysis**) can affect the nail or nail bed. While this type of infection is found in toenails, it can also occur in fingernails.

- Thickened, yellow nail with fungal infection.

Indicators of this slow-growing nail fungal infection may include:

- Debris under the nail
- Nail discoloration
- Nail thickening

Nail Loosening
The nail's open area might have a white appearance where it has separated from the underlying nail bed.

Trauma
Nail trauma can result in nail loosening and even complete nail loss. Nail trauma may occur if:

- A door is slammed into the nail
- Something crushed the nail
- A heavy object is dropped on the nail

Bleeding below the nail could cause enough pressure for the nail to loosen and even fall off. Make sure to reach out to your doctor if you experience nail trauma, especially if there is bleeding.

Shoe Wear
Shoes can cause repeated trauma to your toenails. This may occur while:

THE HUMAN NAIL - Ailments and Diseases
Symptoms, Causes, and Treatment

- Hiking
- Running
- Walking long distances

Taking Part In An Endurance Sport

With trauma, blood may build up beneath the nail and cause red, purple, or black discoloration. It is a **subungual hematoma, jogger's toe,** or **black toenail.** In many cases, you will lose the nail as it grows out.

Repetitive long-term rubbing of the toe against the tip of a shoe may result in the nail edge coming loose without bleeding beneath the nail.

Other Causes

A loose or lifted nail may be caused by:

- A photosensitivity (light sensitivity) response to a medication
- An allergic reaction to manicure/pedicure product
- Hyperthyroidism (thyroid gland is overactive)
- Nail psoriasis with yellow and white discoloration
- Nail psoriasis, a long-term skin condition
- Psoriatic onycholysis
- Treatment for cancer (chemotherapy)

How Do You Treat a Loose Nail?

It is best to see a foot and ankle doctor called a podiatrist or a skin, hair, and nail doctor called a dermatologist to treat a loose nail. Your doctor can diagnose the condition based on its appearance but may also run tests. Treatments will vary depending on the underlying issue.

Your doctor may cut loose nail portions for fungal infections and prescribe anti-fungal medications.

THE HUMAN NAIL - Ailments and Diseases
Symptoms, Causes, and Treatment

You may have to visit an urgent care clinic to drain the blood, cut the nail, or remove the nail for nail trauma. They might also prescribe antibiotics if the nail is infected.

For nail psoriasis, your doctor can give you a topical or oral medication or a steroid injection in the nail.

Regardless of the cause of nail loosening, it is best to seek medical attention as quickly as possible to reduce the possibility of problems.

Will The Nail Grow Back?
After having lost a nail or part of it, you may wonder if your nail will grow back and how it will look. Typically, an exposed nail bed will heal within a few weeks, and the nail will grow back. Still, it could take 12 to 18 months for the nail to grow back, and it may look different.

Treatment for loose fingernails or toenails will vary based on the underlying cause. If you have a loose nail, it is best to reach out to your doctor. They may suggest specific medications or procedures based on your symptoms.

THE HUMAN NAIL - Ailments and Diseases
Symptoms, Causes, and Treatment

Black Toenails

The toenails are white in color. Discolorations may occur from **nail polish, nutritional deficiencies, infection, or trauma.** Black toenails are attributed to various causes, with some resolving themselves. If the nail does not get better, you will need to see a doctor to rule out a more serious cause of black toenails.

What Causes Black Toenails?
A black toenail may be caused by:

- **An underlying medical condition** - including anemia, diabetes, heart disease, or kidney disease.

- **Fungal infection** - while these often look white or yellow, fungal infections can sometimes cause black toenails from debris build-up. Toenails are particularly susceptible to fungal infections because they thrive in moist and warm environments.

- **Melanoma** - this is the most severe skin cancer, which often appears as a dark brown misshapen spot. These spots can also occur underneath nail beds.

- **Trauma** - usually caused by an injury, trauma to the toenail can cause the blood vessels beneath the nail to break. The resulting bleed underneath the nail appears black.

When To See a Doctor

A black toenail does not necessarily require a doctor's visit. The need for treatment depends on the initial cause. Knowing the reason can help you make this decision. On the other side, if you do not see the cause, visiting your doctor is a good idea. Your doctor can diagnose and treat black toenails.

Can a Black Toenail Cause Complications?

Toenail fungus left untreated can spread throughout your feet and other body parts. It can cause lasting nail damage. Complications might also arise from melanoma in the toenail mistaken for trauma-induced black toenail. You need to see your doctor if you notice any black spots spreading throughout the nail or if they do not go away despite your toenail growing out.

What Are The Treatments For Black Toenails?

Fungal infections of the toes can be treated at home when caught early. Over-the-counter ointments, creams, and polishes are usually adequate. Severe cases may require prescription antifungal treatment.

If an injury causes a black toenail, the resulting spot from a broken blood vessel will disappear once the nail grows out. A black toenail caused by trauma from an injury usually resolves without treatment. However, if your toenail grows out and still appears black, the symptoms might be related to another underlying cause. Toenail discoloration associated with diabetes and other health conditions requires treatment for the underlying causes.

What Is The Outlook For a Black Toenail?

The outlook mostly depends on the source of the symptoms. Issues related to trauma and fungal infections have the best outlook. In these cases, injured nails grow out, and fungal infections may be treated at home. Black toenails caused by melanoma, as well as other health conditions, are symptomatic. The outlook for these cases depends on how early you treat the underlying cause.

How To Prevent Black Toenails

Keeping your nails clean and dry can help prevent some causes of the black toenail. You can help prevent toenail trauma by wearing closed-toe shoes when working to prevent the nails from an injury by falling objects. Wearing proper-fitting shoes during a workout (especially running) can help avoid toenail trauma.

It would be best to take other preventive measures regarding additional underlying causes. Decreasing direct sun exposure to your feet and wearing sunscreen around your toes can help prevent melanoma. Black toenails attributed to other medical issues can be prevented through proper treatment and management of the underlying health condition.

THE HUMAN NAIL - Ailments and Diseases
Symptoms, Causes, and Treatment

Brittle Nails

Why Brittle Nails
There can be multiple reasons for easily chipping your nails, such as:

- **Aging** - brittle nails can be a part of the aging process. Along with advancing age, there is a reduction in the moisture content of skin and nails, making them dry.

- **Genetic** - brittle nails can also be due to a congenital disability. It is more likely if your parents also suffer from the same problem.

- **Medical Causes** - anemia, thyroid disorders, diabetes mellitus, poor peripheral circulation during pregnancy, and certain nail disorders like lichen planus, psoriasis, and alopecia areata are other causes of brittleness.

- **Overzealous manicure and pedicure** - inappropriate use of tools during pedicure and manicure like filler, cutter, and especially cuticle makes the nail brittle and more prone to infections.

- **Physical or chemical trauma** - do you use your nails as a tool? Or do you get regular pedicures and manicures?
    - Physical trauma like excessive use of the nail plate in daily chores like opening lids of containers or wearing improper shoes

    - Chemical trauma to the nails in the form of frequent wetting and drying of the hands

    - Exposure to extreme weather and chemicals like detergents, nail polish remover, nail hardeners, hand sanitizers, alkalis, and acids can weaken your nails.

These chemicals damage the protective layer between the cells of a nail

- **Poor nutrition** - deficiency of proteins in the diet can lead to nail chipping because the nail plate is made of keratin. Likewise, biotin deficiency can cause brittle nails, though its role in nail health. Other essential nutrients for nail health are iron, zinc, vitamin C, D, and E.

Brittle Nail Treatments
There are simple brittle nail treatments to remedy the issue, which include:

- **Moisturizers** - are usually meant for the skin, but they also work great for the nails. You can find "super" moisturizing creams to apply to the nails directly.

- **Skip the polish** - if you frequent salons or do not like to have bare fingernails, you could be weakening them, leading to your brittle nail condition. Instead of applying nail color, and removing it with harsh chemicals, go natural and allow your nails to repair themselves.

Clubbing (curved nails)

It is an enlargement of the fingers' ends accompanied by a downward sloping of the nails. Clubbing is also known as **hypertrophic osteoarthropathy (HOA).**

Symptoms of Clubbing
It is typically bilateral (affecting both hands and feet) and should be equal in coverage on both sides.

- **Primary clubbing** - if you or your child has primary HOA, your fingers or toes may naturally appear large, bulging, and rounded. **Primary clubbing is hereditary,** meaning it is passed down via genes. **Congenital clubbing is simply a physical feature,** like the color of your eyes or your height.

- **Secondary clubbing** - happens gradually, and it causes a change in the appearance of the fingers and toes. With secondary clubbing caused by disease, you would also have other features not seen in primary clubbing.

  Features of secondary clubbing include:

  o Disappearing of the angle between the nail and the cuticle
  o Widening or bulging of the distal portion of the finger (where the finger meets the nail)
  o Nail beds that soften and feel spongy
  o Nails that curve downward that look like the bottom of the round part of a spoon
  o Nails that appear to float instead of being firmly attached to the fingers
  o Softening of the nails
  o Warm, red nail beds

- Eventually, the nail and skin about the nail may become shiny, and the nail develops ridging.

Causes of Clubbing

Nail enlargement occurs due to the growth of excess soft tissue beneath the nail beds. **Swelling** is related to inflammation and an increase of small blood vessels in the nail beds. A protein called vascular endothelial growth factor accelerates the growth of blood vessels. This protein is a significant factor in the physical changes in clubbing.

Secondary clubbing occurs as one of the **chronic lung and heart disease effects. Lung cancer is the leading cause of clubbing.** This sign is also associated with several other chronic illnesses, including conditions that involve the thyroid gland or the digestive system.

There are several **health risk factors** associated with secondary clubbing, including:

- An overactive thyroid gland
- Bronchiectasis
- Celiac disease
- Congestive heart failure
- Cyanotic congenital heart disease
- Cystic fibrosis
- Dysentery
- Gastrointestinal neoplasms
- Graves' disease
- Hodgkin lymphoma
- Infective endocarditis
- Inflammatory bowel disease
- Interstitial pulmonary fibrosis
- Liver cirrhosis
- Lung abscess

- Lung cancer
- Other types of cancer, including liver and gastrointestinal
- Pulmonary lymphoma
- Pulmonary tuberculosis

Treatment

The abnormal shape and size of the digits do not cause health problems, but any underlying disease that causes clubbing needs medical management. **Treatments may prevent clubbing from worsening** and, in rare circumstances, may reverse several or all physical characteristics of clubbing.

There are several ways to treat the underlying cause of clubbing, with treatment depending on the situation. You may need respiratory disease management, heart disease treatment, or interventional therapy for cancer.

THE HUMAN NAIL - Ailments and Diseases
Symptoms, Causes, and Treatment

Cracked, Split, Brittle Nails

What Are Cracked Nails?

Healthy nails are smooth, without spots or discoloration. Although they may have vertical ridges, they do not have pits or grooves. Nails that are cracked, split, or brittle may sometimes signify a health problem.

Cracked Nail Causes and Treatments

Aging - the most common reason for cracked nails is getting old. With age, your nails become thinner and more likely to crack. It is most common in women over sixty but may impact men.

If cracked nails are related to aging, you might also see peeling and ridges.

You cannot turn the clock back, so take better care of your nails TODAY. Before bed, put cream or **mineral oil** on your nails and cuticles, and then cotton gloves. During the day, put lotion on after you **wash your hands** or shower. If that is not enough, your dermatologist may be able to prescribe a more substantial treatment.

Harsh nail products - nail polish and nail polish remover can contain strong chemicals. These chemicals will weaken and dry your nails if used often, making them more prone to crack. The adhesives and dyes in acrylic nails can also cause reactions. If nail products are a reason your nails cracked, you may also have:

- Color changes, such as yellowing
- Dull nails

THE HUMAN NAIL - Ailments and Diseases
Symptoms, Causes, and Treatment

Avoid nail products containing toluene and formaldehyde. Both are particularly harsh chemicals. **Biotin**, a B vitamin supplement, can help to heal your nails. But you should not take it if you are **pregnant**.

Note: if your nails are still cracking after six months, see your doctor.

Wet hands - if you spend considerable time with your hands in and out of the **water**, your nails will begin to split. If that is the cause of your cracked nails, you may also have:

- Very soft fingernails
- Cracking is worse in the winter months
- Normal-looking toenails

Lotions with **lanolin** or alpha-hydroxy acid may soothe your nail area. Always wear cotton-lined rubber gloves when your hands are in the water to prevent more splits. Gently file any nail snags or uneven edges, so they do not lead to more cracks.

Psoriasis - the body takes weeks to create new **skin** cells. If it establishes them in just a few days, you have a psoriasis skin condition. It may affect your fingernails and toenails, too. Psoriasis can also cause:

- Tiny pits in the nail bed
- White, yellow, or brown nails
- Loose nails
- Crumbling nails
- Red nail beds

You could have **psoriasis** only on the nails or flaking redness in other places on the body. Visit a dermatologist who can suggest a medicine that helps.

THE HUMAN NAIL - Ailments and Diseases
Symptoms, Causes, and Treatment

Anemia - the body needs iron to make healthy red **blood cells** that can move oxygen to all tissues. Without enough iron, you have **anemia**. Cracked nails can be a symptom.

Pregnancy can increase the chance of **anemia**. So can conditions like **ulcers** and **cancer**. Other symptoms of iron deficiency are:

- **Fatigue**
- Shortness of breath
- Pale skin
- Cold hands and **feet**
- Sore, **swollen tongue**
- Cracks on the sides of your **mouth**

If you think you have anemia, speak to your doctor to determine what is causing it. You might have to take **iron supplements**.

Thyroid disease - the **thyroid** is a gland in your neck. It makes hormones that control many things the body does, like **breathing** and **heart rate**. If the thyroid does not produce sufficient hormones, you suffer from **hypothyroidism**. If this is the reason for your cracked nails, you could also have:

- Brittle nails that break off
- Swelling in your lower legs
- Swelling around your **eyes**
- **Itchy skin**
- **Thinning hair** or bald patches
- Yellow-orange skin on the palms or the soles of your feet
- A doughy or swollen face

If you have some of the above indicators, talk with your doctor. A simple blood test may check how well your thyroid is working.

Note: if your thyroid is the problem, you will have to take a pill every day to provide your body with the hormone your thyroid can no longer make.

THE HUMAN NAIL - Ailments and Diseases
Symptoms, Causes, and Treatment

Fungal infection - yeast or mold can enter your nail and cause an infection, making your nails more likely to crack or break. A fungal infection is more common in the toenails than in your fingernails. You may hear your doctor call the infection **onychomycosis.**

Fungal infections can also produce:

- Nails that are yellow, brown, or white
- Thick nails
- Nails that separate from the bed

Fungal infections can be challenging to treat. Your doctor will give you a prescription for antifungal pills. In severe cases, they might have to take off the nail.

Biotin deficiency - is rare, but you could have cracked nails because you do not have sufficient biotin in your diet. Other symptoms of biotin insufficiency are:

- Hair thinning or loss
- A red rash around the eyes, nose, or mouth
- Pinkeye (conjunctivitis)
- Depression
- Less energy

Biotin supplements can help. You could also try eating more meat, eggs, fish, seeds, nuts, and vegetables like sweet potatoes.

Ingrown Toenails

An ingrown toenail can result from incorrect nail trimming, which includes cutting the toenails too short and tapering the corners to match the curves of the toe. The big toe is more likely to get an ingrown toenail of all the toes. You can treat ingrown toenails at home. However, if your toenail has punctured the skin or if there is any sign of infection, seek medical treatment.

Signs of infection include:

- Pus
- Redness and swelling
- Warmth

What Causes Ingrown Toenails?

Ingrown toenails take place in both men and women. They are more common in people with sweaty feet, such as teenagers. Older people may also be at a higher risk because the toenails thicken with age.

Many issues can cause an ingrown toenail, including:

- Cutting toenails incorrectly? Just cut straight across since angling the sides of the nail can encourage the nail to grow into the skin.

- Shoes placing pressure on the big toes, like socks, stockings, and shoes that are too tight, narrow, or flat for your feet

- Genetic predisposition

THE HUMAN NAIL - Ailments and Diseases
Symptoms, Causes, and Treatment

- Inadequate foot hygiene, such as not keeping your feet clean or dry

- Irregular, curved toenails

- Poor posture

- Toenail injury, including bumping your toe, dropping something heavy on your foot, or kicking a ball repeatedly

Using the feet extensively during athletic activities can make you prone to getting ingrown toenails. Behaviors in which you repeatedly kick an object or put pressure on your feet for prolonged periods can cause toenail damage and increase the risk of ingrown toenails. These activities may include:

- Ballet
- Football
- Kickboxing
- Soccer

What Are The Symptoms Of Ingrown Toenails?
Your toe may become stiff, swollen, and tender in the early stages. It may become red, infected, and very sore, and pus might drain from it as it progresses. Eventually, the skin on the sides of the toenail might start to grow over the nail. Ingrown toenails may be painful, and they usually worsen in stages.

If the toe becomes infected, symptoms may include:

- Bleeding
- Foul smell
- Oozing pus discharge
- Overgrowth of skin around the toe

- Pain
- Red, swollen skin
- Swelling
- Warm to the touch

Stages of Ingrown Toenail Severity

- Stage 1 - the nail has grown into the skin, causing pain and inflammation.

- Stage 2 - new, inflamed tissue grows around the edges of the ingrown toenail. It can lead to drainage or pus.

- Stage 3 - the skin surrounding the toenail is chronically inflamed and secreting pus. Swollen tissue begins to grow over the nail

Treat an ingrown toenail as early as possible to avoid additional symptoms. Never try to cut out an ingrown toenail on your own. It can be excruciating and lead to a severe infection.

How Are Ingrown Toenails Diagnosed?
Your doctor may diagnose your toe with a physical exam. If the toe is infected, you will need an X-ray to show how deep the nail has grown into the skin. The X-ray will also reveal if an ingrown nail has been caused by injury.

Treatment For Ingrown Toenail
Treatment can include:

- Prescribing antibiotics
- Surgery to cut off a part of the nail (partial nail avulsion)
- Trimming the ingrown section of the nail

Surgical Treatment

There are several kinds of surgical treatments for ingrown toenails. Partial nail removal only involves removing the portion of the nail that is digging into the skin. Your doctor will numb the toe and then narrows the toenail. According to, partial nail removal is 98 percent effective for preventing future ingrown toenails.

In partial nail removal, the sides of the nail are excised so that the sides are completely straight. A bit of cotton is set under the residual portion of the nail to keep the ingrown toenail from recurring. Your doctor can also treat your toe with phenol, which keeps the nail from growing back.

Total nail removal may be utilized when the ingrown nail is caused by thickening. Your doctor gives you a local pain injection and then removes the entire nail in a procedure called a matrixectomy.

After surgery - your surgeon will send you home with your toe bandaged. You will need to keep your foot raised for one to two days, have daily saltwater soaks until your toe heals, and wear an open-toe shoe allowing your toe to heal correctly. The dressing is usually removed two days after surgery. Your doctor will prescribe pain relief medication and antibiotics to prevent infection. Avoid unnecessary movement during this healing process.

The toenail will grow back a few months after a partial nail removal surgery. If the entire nail is removed to the base, the toenail can take over a year to grow back.

Complications of ingrown toenails - if left untreated, an ingrown toenail infection can result in an infection of the bone in the toe. A toenail infection may also cause foot ulcers, open sores, and a loss of blood flow in the infected area. Tissue decomposition and tissue death at the site of infection are possible.

Feet infections may be more severe if you have diabetes. Even a slight cut, scrape, or ingrown toenails can promptly become infected due to a lack of blood circulation and nerve sensitivity. Visit your doctor immediately if you are diabetic and concerned about an ingrown nail infection.

When you have a genetic predisposition to ingrown toenails, they can come back or reappear on several toes at once. Your quality of life can be affected by infections and other painful foot issues that require multiple treatments or surgeries. Your doctor may recommend a partial or complete matrixectomy to remove the toenails causing chronic pain in such circumstances.

THE HUMAN NAIL - Ailments and Diseases
Symptoms, Causes, and Treatment

Koilonychia (spoon-shaped nails)

What Is Koilonychia
The name Koilonychia refers to **soft nails with a spoon-shaped dent in them.** Often spoon nails form gradually, and the first indication is flattened nails in many people. Eventually, an indentation will start, which can be deep enough to hold a drop of water on the nail bed.

Symptoms Of Koilonychia
You may not have enough iron if you have thin fingernails that dip down in the middle and look like spoons. An iron deficiency can be explained for numerous reasons, such as:

- Lack of proper nutrition
- A health problem in the stomach or intestines
- Sensitivity to gluten (celiac disease)
- High altitude

Causes Of Koilonychia
Iron deficiency (the world's most common nutritional deficiency disease) is the most frequent cause of koilonychia. It commonly affects children and women of childbearing age.

Note: Koilonychia is a symptom, not an infection. But some people with fungal nail infections can also get spoon nails.

Genetic factors - Koilonychia can occur as a result of some genetic conditions. Which can involve:

- **Hemochromatosis** - absorbs too much iron from the diet.
- **Nail-patella syndrome** - problems with the nails, kneecaps, hip bones, and elbows.

THE HUMAN NAIL - Ailments and Diseases
Symptoms, Causes, and Treatment

Koilonychia may be an indication that you may have:

- Cancer
- Heart disease
- Hypothyroidism
- Iron-deficiency anemia
- Lupus erythematosus is an autoimmune disease that triggers inflammation
- Raynaud's disease, a condition limiting blood circulation

Note: Koilonychia is not always a symptom of an underlying disease. One can have spoon nails due to an injury or overexposure to petroleum products. For example, hairstylists use petroleum products routinely for specific hair treatments.

Treatment Of Koilonychia (podiatrist or dermatologist)
If you have an iron deficiency, changing your diet or taking supplements may correct and prevent spoon nails. Eat more iron-rich foods, such as:

- Beans and lentils
- Dark chocolate
- Fortified foods, such as bread or breakfast cereal
- Iron-rich fruit, such as dates, figs, prunes, and raisins
- Leafy greens, like spinach or kale
- Meat and seafood rich in iron
- Nuts and seeds

Note: often, treating the underlying cause of koilonychia will help the nails grow correctly. But it can take a long time (six to 18 months).

THE HUMAN NAIL - Ailments and Diseases
Symptoms, Causes, and Treatment

Nail Fungus

These infections can be spread from person to person and affect the fingernails and toenails. Without treatment, the nail bed can become infected. Those with diabetes or compromised immune systems have a higher risk of fungal infection.

What Is Nail Fungus
A fungal nail infection will occur when a fungus penetrates a person's nail, usually through a small crack. Fungal nail infections occur more frequently on toenails than fingernails.

Symptoms Of Nail Fungus
Fungal nail infections include:

- Crumbling of the nail plate
- Discoloration, usually in streaks
- Distorted nail
- Flaking white areas on the nail's surface
- Lifting the nail plate off of the nail bed
- Scaling under the nails
- Thickened or brittle nail
- Treatments
- White or yellow streaks on the nail
- White, yellow, or green smelly discharge
- Yellow spots at the lower end of the nail

Causes Of Nail Fungus
A dermatophyte fungus is a cause. Yeast and molds can also cause nail fungus. If nail discoloration is detected, the nail may sometimes have a white spot or turn yellow, brown, or green. Oral antifungal medication is generally used. Antifungal nail

lacquer or a topical solution can be effective. Also, the medicine will vary depending on the type and extent of infection.

Causes of fungal nail infections include:

- A weak immune system
- Athlete's foot
- Circulation problems
- Diabetes
- Nail injury

Treatment Of Nail Fungus (dermatologist)
Doctors can treat fungal nail infections with antifungal pills or surgically remove the nail.

Self-care

- Do not wear the same shoes.
- Keep feet dry and clean to resist fungal growth, and use an antifungal foot powder in shoes and socks.
- Make sure shoes are of the correct size.

Medication
Oral antifungals - such as terbinafine (Lamisil) or fluconazole (Diflucan), are usually used to treat toenail fungus. These treatments are effective, but they may cause serious side effects ranging from gastrointestinal problems, dizziness, severe skin problems, and jaundice.

Topical antifungals - several over-the-counter (OTC) treatments are available to treat nail fungus in liquids, solutions, and creams. These products are applied directly to the nail and surrounding skin to treat cases of nail fungus infection. Common topical antifungals include clotrimazole and terbinafine.

THE HUMAN NAIL - Ailments and Diseases
Symptoms, Causes, and Treatment

Note: OTC products such as terbinafine cream may provide relief in conjunction with regular debridement and consistent use over four to six months.

Nail-Patella Syndrome

Nail patella syndrome (NPS), sometimes called Fong syndrome or hereditary osteoonychodysplasia (HOOD), is a **rare genetic disorder.**

What Is Nail Patella Syndrome
An uncommon genetic mutation that affects an estimated 1 in 50,000 people. It causes **changes in nails, kneecaps, hip bones, and elbows. The most widespread symptom of the syndrome is underdeveloped or missing fingernails and toenails.**

Symptoms Of Nail Patella
The following are some symptoms of this rare condition:

- Discolored nails
- Knee and elbow pain
- Missing fingernails and toenails
- Ridged or split fingernails and toenails
- Small bony growths on hip bones (iliac horns)
- Small, deformed, or missing kneecaps
- Underdeveloped fingernails and toenails
- Underdeveloped or deformed elbows

Causes Of Nail Patella
A genetic mutation causes nail patella.

Treatment Of Nail Patella
None

Nail Pitting

If you have dents in the nails that look like an ice pick made them, this could signify that you have a disease that affects your entire body.

Health disorders that may lead to the development of nail pitting include:

- **Alopecia areata** - an autoimmune disease that causes the immune system to attack hair follicles

- **Atopic and contact dermatitis** - types of eczema that can cause itchiness, rash, and bumps on the skin

- **Incontinentia pigmenti** - a genetic condition that causes skin abnormalities like a blistering rash, wart-like skin growths, and gray or brown patches

- **Lichen planus** - an autoimmune disease that causes inflammation on the skin and inside the mouth

- **Nail problems associated with psoriasis**

- **Pemphigus Vulgaris** - a rare group of autoimmune diseases that cause blisters on the skin and mucous membranes

- **Reactive arthritis** - a form of arthritis that develops due to an infection

- **Sarcoidosis** - an inflammatory disease that affects multiple organs

Treatment Of Nail Pitting

For mild cases of nail pitting, treatment is not required. It is especially true if the nail pitting does not cause any discomfort. Medicinal creams are not always effective since they may not reach the nail bed. However, in some cases, nail pitting can be treated with vitamin D3 and a corticosteroid, a drug that can help reduce inflammation.

Preventing Nail Pitting

There is no way to prevent nail pitting. Still, some things can prevent it from worsening.

To keep your nails healthy:

- Avoid specific triggers of an existing skin disorder, such as smoking, alcohol use, and obesity
- Avoid getting manicures because they can damage your nails further
- Eat a diet abundant in vitamins and nutrients
- Keep your nails short
- Stay hydrated
- Use a moisturizer on your hands and feet to keep your skin hydrated
- Wear gloves if you work with your hands

THE HUMAN NAIL - Ailments and Diseases
Symptoms, Causes, and Treatment

Nail Psoriasis

According to the **National Psoriasis Foundation,** roughly 50% of individuals with psoriasis have nail psoriasis. **Nail psoriasis may affect a person's fingernails or toenails.**

What Is Nail Psoriasis?
People living with psoriasis may develop symptoms. It occurs when psoriasis affects the skin of the nail bed or near the nail beds. Most treatment options for split nails are home remedies. In most cases, nails will split because of repeated drying and wetting, leading to dryness and brittleness. The effects can be even harsher in the winter with dry heat or in areas with low humidity. The recommended solution is to apply lotions with lanolin or alpha-hydroxy acids after soaking the nails in water for five minutes or more.

Symptoms Of Nail Psoriasis
Symptoms will vary depending on the type. Common symptoms include:

- A build-up of debris beneath the nail
- Crumbling nails
- Nail pitting, in which tiny dents appear in the nail
- Nail ridges
- Nail thickening
- Pain or tenderness
- Separation of the nail from a finger or toe
- The blood beneath the nail
- White, yellow, or brown discoloration

Causes Of Nail Psoriasis

Experts believe the exact cause of psoriasis is a combination of health issues. Something is wrong with the immune system causing inflammation and triggering new skin cells to form too quickly. Generally, skin cells are replaced every 10 to 30 days. But with psoriasis, new cells grow every 3 to 4 days, leaving behind a buildup of the old cells replaced by the new ones.

Things that could trigger an outbreak of psoriasis are:

- Cuts, scrapes, or surgery
- Emotional stress
- Strep infections
- Medications, including blood pressure medications, anti-malarial drugs, lithium, mood stabilizers, antibiotics, and NSAIDs

Treatment Of Nail Psoriasis (dermatologist)

Nail psoriasis can be treated by:

- calcipotriol, to treat build-up under the nail
- injections of corticosteroids
- strong corticosteroid cream
- tazarotene, to treat pitting and discoloration

These topical medications can be over-the-counter or prescription and come in various forms, such as:

- creams
- emulsions
- nail polishes
- ointments

Nail psoriasis may be challenging to treat and may require more than one type of treatment. If more potent treatments are needed, a dermatologist might attempt:

- Applying corticosteroids next to the nails
- Laser treatment
- PUVA is a therapy that involves exposing nails to UVA rays after immersing them in psoralen
- Using medications to treat both skin and nail psoriasis

Is There a Cure?
There is no cure, but treatment dramatically reduces symptoms, even in severe cases. **When you control the inflammation of psoriasis, the risk of heart disease, stroke, metabolic syndrome, and other diseases associated with inflammation diminishes.**

THE HUMAN NAIL - Ailments and Diseases
Symptoms, Causes, and Treatment

Onychoschizia (nail ridges)

When looking at your fingernails, you may be able to make out faint raised lines running vertically (aligned with the fingers) or horizontally (across the nails). Occasionally, especially when these ridges are very defined and apparent, they can cause your fingernails to look abnormal. **Vertical ridges are considered a genetic attribute to one's fingernails and do not always require alarm or treatment. Horizontal lines are more serious, directly indicating an underlying medical condition.**

What is Onychoschizia?

The condition known as Onychoschizia happens when **vertical ridges form on the nails.** Typically, the surface of a person's nails is very smooth, but for anyone who suffers from Onychoschizia, the nails' **surfaces become rough, and scales tend to develop.** The conditions of Onychoschizia can be on all the nails of a person or can be limited to only one or two nails.

Onychoschizia **is not a dangerous disease but may be related to the signs of some nutritional deficiencies in the body of the person suffering from it.** Various treatments are available online and from your doctor.

Symptoms Of Onychoschizia

Many people have ridges and lines on their nails. Especially individuals involved in rigorous and heavy work such as construction or any other occupation that includes extensive use of their hands. Ridging starts at the joint from wear. The condition is found in individuals **deficient in vitamins and minerals, as their nails are fragile and lack the components that give strength and luster.**

Occasionally, it is possible that the ridging is only present on one finger rather than all the fingers. It happens when the person has suffered from any injury or has crushed that nail under some weight. So, **onychoschizia** tends to develop in that fingernail. In some instances, the process of ridging will be followed by brittle nails, which can split at the ends slightly.

**Causes Of Onychoschizia
Vertical Fingernail Ridges:**

- **Loss of Moisture** - age will also affect the appearance of the nails. As you get older, the nails begin to lose their moisture which causes fingernail ridges. The aging process has a damaging impact on nails, pulling away moisture rather than providing it. The skin dehydrates more quickly, causing the nail beds to lose natural oils to keep the nails smooth.

- **Malabsorption** - sometimes, our bodies may inadvertently work against us. When you eat plenty of protein, calcium, and vitamin-rich foods, but your fingernails display deep ridges, it might mean that your body has **nutrient absorption issues.** It is essential to consult a doctor to determine what is going on in this situation. It is crucial to find out what is causing your malabsorption because you may need **medical treatments or prescription medications** to help resolve the issues.

- **Malnutrition** - what foods do you eat regularly, and what foods are missing from your meals? Certain foods such as lean meats, fresh vegetables, and whole fruits contain essential vitamins and nutrients that the body needs to be healthy. **If you have a deficiency in protein, iron, calcium, or vitamins A or B, this can trigger abnormal ridges in your nails.**

Horizontal Fingernail Ridges

Diets lacking essential nutrients can disrupt the keratin formation in your nails and cause horizontal lines. Inadequate moisture produces nail ridges and can make the nails brittle and prone to breakage. **Horizontal ridges are also caused by respiratory diseases, autoimmune diseases, skin disorders, and exposure to harsh toxins.**

- **Beau's Lines** - are characterized by deep, linear grooves and cells that have been darkened underneath the nail. These lines indicate trauma, chemotherapy, malnutrition, acute illnesses, and metabolic problems. All of these disorders cause interruptions in the protein synthesized by the nail.
  Other conditions which cause Beau's lines:
  - Diseases that cause high fever, such as measles, mumps, and scarlet fever
  - Peripheral vascular disease
  - Pneumonia
  - Uncontrolled diabetes
  - Zinc deficiency

- **Familiarize Yourself With The Different Types of Horizontal Fingernail Ridges** - transverse ridges indicate a history of severe illnesses. If you have suffered from threatening diseases or a terminal illness, such as cancer, these ridges will appear on your nails.

- **Mee's Lines** - can appear as transverse white lines across the nails. Arsenic poisoning or poisoning due to other heavy, toxic materials causes these lines to appear.

- **Muehrcke Lines** - appear when there is a disruption in the pigmentation of the nail. Kidneys and liver disease, malnutrition, and chemotherapy are associated with causing these kinds of horizontal lines on the nails.

THE HUMAN NAIL - Ailments and Diseases
Symptoms, Causes, and Treatment

- **Onychotillomania (washboard nails)** - if there are grooves and ridges in the **center of your thumbnails**, you might have developed a habit of picking at (or pushing back) the cuticles on your nails. Many people are not aware that they do this.

- **Terry's Nails** - are characterized by having a white nail plate. Someone with Terry's nails will also have a dark horizontal band at the tip of the nail. Those with diabetes, HIV, kidney disorders, or liver disease can have Terry's nails.

- **Transverse Ridges** - are indicative of a history of severe illness. These ridges will appear on your nails if you suffer consistently threatening diseases or a terminal illness, such as cancer.

Onychoschizia Is Due To Many Reasons
Some of the most common reasons are:

- Amyloidosis, an excessive protein build-up in the individual's body, can cause onychoschizia.

- Eczema can be a reason behind onychoschizia. In this condition, the area surrounding the nails becomes soft and loses its strength, making the nail lose.

- Exposure to certain chemicals and excessive moisture can lead to the problem of onychoschizia. Chemicals tend to make nails weaker and more prone to breaking.

- If a person has an excessive nail biting or finger chewing habit, this tends to weaken the nails and give rise to the condition of onychoschizia.

- In females, the disorder of onychoschizia is more common due to using **nail polish remover, which weakens the nail and makes the layers of the nail thin.** Consequently, the nail becomes more susceptible to breakage.

- Sometimes, an individual's eating habits give rise to a disorder like onychoschizia. It is due to **unhealthy food habits** or an **excessive intake of specific vitamins or minerals.**

Onychoschizia Treatment (dermatologists)

Onychoschizia is a disorder that does not require any particular kind of treatment or attention. It usually occurs as a side effect or the normal aging process. However, if one finds that their nails have become brittle and are naturally breaking away, they may follow the easy treatments for curing the problem of onychoschizia.

THE HUMAN NAIL - Ailments and Diseases
Symptoms, Causes, and Treatment

Onychogryphosis (ram's horn nails)

A nail disease causes one side of the nail to grow more quickly than others. The nickname for this malady is **ram's horn nails** since nails are thick and curvy, like horns or claws. Onychogryphosis primarily affects the toes, specifically the big toe.

If you suffer from onychogryphosis, your nails will appear:

- Curved
- Long (extending beyond the toe)
- Unusually thick
- Yellow or brown

Ram's horn nails can develop at different ages depending on the underlying cause. It can be especially problematic for young and older adults. If you think you have onychogryphosis, seek treatment. The condition will get worse over time and can also cause:

- Inability to engage in physical activities like sports or physically active careers
- Infection
- Ingrown nails
- Pain
- Time away from work

Causes Of Onychogryphosis
The following are known causes of onychogryphosis

- **Foot trauma** - repeatedly hurting your feet or minor foot trauma can damage the toes and nail plates, eventually leading to onychogryphosis. For example, wearing tight or too small shoes will result in foot trauma.

Onychogryphosis may also develop if you have a condition like hammertoe. Treatment may be as simple as wearing shoes of the correct size. You could also use splints and pads to train the toes and nails to grow normally.

- **Fungal infection** - onychomycosis is a fungal infection that causes the **nails to become thick, crinkly, and brittle.** This infection primarily affects toenails but can also impact fingernails. Doctors diagnose onychomycosis by examining the skin tissue swabbed or scraped from beneath an affected nail. Oral or topical antibiotics may be used for treating fungal infections.

- **Psoriasis** - is **a common autoimmune disease** that makes the body generate extra skin cells. These cells build up and form red, dry, scaly patches of skin. The skin growths can also affect the nails. Almost half of the people with psoriasis experience nail changes. **One-third of people with nail psoriasis also have onychomycosis.** Steroid injections into the nail beds may be able to treat these growths. Taking antifungal medication may also help. If treatments do not work, you will need surgery.

- **Peripheral vascular disease** - also called **peripheral artery disease (PAD),** causes the arteries in the legs to build up with plaque. It reduces blood flow in the legs and feet, and you may notice sores due to improper blood flow and slow or abnormal nail growth. If untreated, PAD can lead to onychogryphosis. **Smoking is the leading risk factor in developing PAD.** Options for treatment include lifestyle changes, medication, and surgery to clear the artery of plaque.

- **Ichthyosis - is a rare skin condition that excludes the body from getting rid of dead skin cells.** Common symptoms of this genetic condition are **thickened or deformed nails, which can turn into onychogryphosis** in some cases. Ichthyosis is diagnosed when babies are born with a collodion membrane on the skin. Topical creams or oral retinoids are the most common treatment methods. If onychogryphosis develops, surgery may be necessary.

- **Tuberous sclerosis complex (TSC) - is a rare genetic disease that causes benign tumors to grow throughout the body.** TSC is typically diagnosed because of skin problems, including nail deformities. Though the nail deformities go away in some cases, they may worsen, turning them into ram's horn nails. **Additional symptoms of TSC include cognitive impairment, autism, and seizures.** Treatment for ram's horn nails that are related to TSC is surgery.

Treatment Of Onychogryphosis
Surgery is the sole treatment option for onychogryphosis. However, the type and frequency of the surgery are based on the cause of the ram's horn nails. If this condition is genetic, you may have to get the same surgery multiple times as the nails grow back. Your doctor may suggest permanently removing the affected nail plate to solve this problem.

If the cause is less severe, like foot trauma or infection, your doctor will perform surgery to correct the problem. They will then teach you how to cut your nails and care for your feet properly, so the issue does not occur again. Toenails must be clipped straight across rather than curved to help avoid ingrown nails. Always wear clean cotton socks that can absorb moisture and help prevent fungal infections. Additional treatment methods may address the underlying cause of ram's horn nails to prevent the condition from developing.

Managing Ram's Horn Nails

Ram's horn nails are unsightly, but they are also painful and can severely impact your quality of life.

While not always possible to prevent onychogryphosis, the following are a few simple things you can do to promote nail health:

- Change socks regularly
- Cut toenails straight rather than curved at the edges
- Keep nails trimmed short
- Wear cotton socks that absorb moisture
- Wear gloves when handling chemicals
- Wear shoes that fit and that have room in the toe area

You can manage ram's horn nails by:

- Regular visits to your foot doctor
- Use a wheelchair or motorized scooter to keep pressure off the feet
- Wearing adaptive shoes

Onycholysis (loose nails)

A loose toenail or fingernail could be a troubling symptom, especially if you do not know what caused it. Getting a loose nail is a process that impacts only part of the nail. However, if there has been trauma to the nail, the entire nail can come loose quickly in some instances. **Onycholysis can occur in the fingernails or toenails.**

What Is Onycholysis?
Onycholysis is when an individual's **nail or nails detach from the skin underneath.** Although not a critical health condition, onycholysis can be a symptom of a potentially severe illness.

It is crucial to understand what onycholysis is and what it may mean so that you can make informed medical decisions.

Though not always possible to prevent onycholysis. You can:

- Avoiding wearing warm, damp shoes for prolonged periods

- Eat a balanced diet while supplementing with vitamin D and iron if needed

- Keeping psoriasis under control with therapies and medications

- Managing any thyroid conditions

- Wear gloves and appropriate footwear when exercising or performing manual labor

THE HUMAN NAIL - Ailments and Diseases
Symptoms, Causes, and Treatment

Symptoms Of Onycholysis
When a person has onycholysis, **the nail will pull away from the nail bed beneath.** The person may also notice that **the nail turns a different color.** The color that it changes to depends on what is causing the onycholysis.

Some of the possible colors include:

- Gray
- Green
- Purple
- White
- Yellowish

Onycholysis is in itself not painful. Nevertheless, the underlying cause of onycholysis may cause pain.

Causes Of Onycholysis
The cause of onycholysis varies. But most commonly, a person may experience an injury or repetitive trauma.

Some other typical causes include:

- An allergic reaction
- An infection
- Certain cancer treatments
- Footwear
- Fungal infections, common in the feet
- Health conditions
- Psoriasis
- Reactions to chemicals, such as nail polish, nail polish remover, or household cleaners
- Reaction to medication
- Trauma

THE HUMAN NAIL - Ailments and Diseases
Symptoms, Causes, and Treatment

If a nail detaches from the nail bed, it could be a medical issue. One of the usual suspects in the above list may be the first symptom of something more serious inside the body if onycholysis cannot be explained.

Health problems that can cause onycholysis can consist of:

- A yeast infection
- A thyroid disorder
- Vitamin and mineral deficiencies

Treatment Of Onycholysis
Step one in treating onycholysis is determining what is causing the nail to lift. Treating the proper condition will allow the nail to heal and reattach to the skin as it grows out again.

Injuries may not require much additional treatment. However, if the skin is open, it is essential to keep the area clean and prevent infection. Be careful in cleaning under the nail, as water could push bacteria or fungus deeper beneath the nail.

Fungal Infections require antifungal medications to heal the underlying infection. Fungal medications are dispensed through medicated creams and ointments applied next to or on the nail.

- Psoriasis is a chronic skin condition indicated by red, scaly patches on the skin. In some cases, psoriasis can affect the nails, turning an ashy color and detaching from the nail bed underneath. Psoriasis is typically treated with topical creams, biologics, systemic, or phototherapy.

- Thyroid problems can cause onycholysis and often require medications that help the thyroid regulate hormone production.

- Dietary changes most frequently treat vitamin and mineral deficiencies. In some instances, a doctor will prescribe or advise supplements. An individual with brittle or detaching nails may be required to take iron supplements to help the nails regain strength.

Home treatments that might improve onycholysis include a variety of essential oils. Evidence exists that tea tree oil may help treat fungus infections. Tea tree oil, combined with a carrier oil, have natural antifungal properties that might mean an individual does not have to seek further treatment.

Whatever the cause, it is important to follow the doctor's instructions on treating the underlying condition. Failure to treat the underlying cause may result in onycholysis worsening or recurring.

Onychomycosis (thick toenails)

What Are Thick Toenails?
Changes in the toenails may be a symptom of an underlying condition. Toenails that grow thicker over time indicate a **fungal infection** known as onychomycosis. If not treated, thick toenails can become painful. Prompt treatment can be vital to curing the nail fungus. **Fungal infections might be difficult to heal and may require months of treatment.**

What Symptoms Accompany Thick Toenails?
Changes in the thickness of toenails may be just one symptom of a fungal infection. Other symptoms of nail fungus include:

- A foul smell that comes from the toenail
- Toenails that can lift from the nail bed
- Toenails that vary in color to yellow, brown, or green
- Toenails that look scaly or chalky
- Toenails that split or crumble
- Toenails with dirt under them

You may not notice any discomfort in the early stages of the infection. But, as symptoms build, your toenails may become painful.

What Causes Thick Toenails?
Around 1 to 8 percent of the population is diagnosed with onychomycosis. This condition can occur when a fungus or yeast enters your toenail:

- From a crack in the toenails
- From a cut in your skin that touches your toenail
- Where your toenail and nail bed meet

THE HUMAN NAIL - Ailments and Diseases
Symptoms, Causes, and Treatment

The fungus or yeast will grow under the nail bed, which is moist. The infection is initially minor but may spread and cause your toenail to grow thicker, which leads to other symptoms. Toes are susceptible to fungal infections because of their exposure to wet areas.

Who Is At Risk For Getting Thick Toenails?
You can get toenail fungus from:

- Athlete's foot that spreads to your toenails
- Being barefoot in public places, like swimming pools, showers, and gyms
- Damage to a toenail
- Frequent or prolonged exposure to water
- Genetics
- Medications that suppress your immune system
- Shoes that constrict your feet
- Smoking
- Sweaty feet and shoes

You might get a toenail fungus if you have an existing medical condition, like:

- Type 1 diabetes
- Type 2 diabetes
- Circulatory conditions
- Psoriasis

Cancer treatments can increase the likelihood of developing nail fungus. If you have an existing condition and develop fungus, it is crucial to treat it immediately.

How Are Thick Toenails Diagnosed?
Call your doctor if you observe a change in the appearance of your nails. Treating a fungal infection as soon as possible helps prevent the condition from worsening. Your doctor will look at the nails to diagnose the condition and may swab under the nail or take a toenail clipping to confirm the condition.

Can Thick Toenails Cause Complications?
Untreated toenail infections can cause some complications. Over time, the condition may worsen, and symptoms can become more severe. The toenails might thicken to the point that they cause discomfort when wearing shoes or even make walking more challenging. If you have preexisting medical conditions, treatment will be vital so that the fungus does not add secondary infections and impediments.

How Are Thick Toenails Treated?
Not all cases of toenail fungus need medical treatment. Thick toenails can be a symptom of a worsening fungus. Try home-based therapies first, and then talk to your doctor about prescription-based options if unsuccessful.

Medical Treatments
Toenail fungus can require medical interventions that involve prescriptions and recommendations from your doctor. These include:

- Laser treatments
- Oral medications
- Elimination of the toenail to treat the nail bed
- Topical medications

If you are taking oral medication prescriptions, you may need routine blood testing, as some of these medications can affect the liver.

Note: you can experience a recurrence of toenail fungus after treatment. Inform your doctor if you experience chronic fungal infections.

Can Thick Toenails Be Prevented?

You can reduce the risk of thick toenails and the recurrence of toenail fungus in several ways:

- Buy new footwear after your nail fungus is cured

- Groom your feet properly

- Keep feet clean by washing them with soap and water daily. Dry them off with a towel afterward

- Keep feet as dry as possible. Change socks a few times a day, wear cotton socks that remove moisture from the feet, rotate shoes so they can dry out, and purchase shoes that breathe. Do not constrict your feet.

- Use a foot powder that keeps your feet dry

- Use disinfected tools when trimming your nails

- Wear flip-flops or other shower shoes in locker rooms or at the pool

Onychophosis (callus build-up)

Callus build-up (onychophosis) is a local or spread-out thickening of the outer layer of skin that builds upon the side or central nail folds from the nail folds to the nail plate. A common problem in older people, onychophosis, can include a hematoma directly due to recurring minor injury and usually tends to affect the 1st and 5th toes.

Calluses can build up as a defensive action on the border of the sulcus. It could be expanded to a level where even minor tension to the nail plate or the sulcus wall can increase severe discomfort. There can be connected hypertrophy of the shoulders of the nail plate, and the areas affected will need to be removed and remedied with compounds that soften keratin. Although uncomfortable, they never feel painful as ingrown toenails do. The nail is not wedged into the skin layers in this particular disorder. However, a little bump under the skin expands in the narrow channel of the epidermis alongside the nail and underneath the nail and can be very unpleasant.

Causes Of Onychophosis
More than one nail and its adjoining soft skin changes, nail fold increasing could be the main reasons behind onychomycosis. Some other triggers could be a recurring minor injury and inappropriate footwear, which could be making contributions.

Moving the feet can result in rubbing the big toes' outer skin and the inside skin of the big toe when hard-pressed against the second toe. The rubbing can also appear on smaller toes and displays an accumulation of rigid skin on the sides of the nails.

Treatment Of Onychophosis (podiatrist or dermatologist)
Callus reduction is straightforward and rarely requires a local anesthetic. The bumps in or under the skin are without nerves, so they can be trimmed away without discomfort.

A few treatment solutions can deal with onychophosis and may involve nail softeners, nail packing, and, if necessary, removal. Tough skin layers beneath the nail soften, resulting in a simple excision of the keratinous substance without discomfort. The affected person is recommended to use a nail softener daily but modestly, with a single drop on each impacted region.

The only noticeable complication is yellowing in the region, which does not negatively impact you. Do not use this treatment on infected or sore areas, and it is not for those with poor blood flow and diabetic issues. Recurrences can be stopped by wearing suitable footwear to reduce the pressure of the nail plate on adjoining nail folds.

Onychophosis surgical treatment includes a sensible scalpel method to scrape the callus thoroughly to clean the edge of the nail from the sulci. For skin thickening of soft tissues like onychophosis, the primary therapy is removing dead skin with a sterile blade and keeping away from any blood loss. Toe separators can protect the inner portion of the big toe. Increasing foot functionality through training and orthotic modification can decrease the rubbing. In more complicated conditions, surgical elimination of the side of the nail could enable the sulci additional room. If the skin fails to contact the side of the toe, it cannot develop a callus.

THE HUMAN NAIL - Ailments and Diseases
Symptoms, Causes, and Treatment

Onychoschizia (split nails)

Split nails are usually caused by physical stress, nutrient deficiency, or wear and tear. Split nails can be a problem, primarily if you work with your hands. However, split nails are entirely normal and sometimes unavoidable. In some instances, one can take precautionary measures to prevent splitting their nails. In other circumstances, splitting a nail may be inevitable.

Split nails can affect fingernails and toenails and are typically a result of physical trauma. Wear and tear, in addition to nutrient deficiencies, are also possible causes. A split can occur vertically or horizontally across the nail.

Causes Of Onychoschizia

A split nail is characterized by a **crack starting in the nail.** This issue is usually due to vitamin deficiencies or internal diseases in rare situations, with iron deficiency being the most common cause. Nail splitting is caused by low specific proteins, folic acid, or vitamin C levels.

Other causes of split nails include:

- **Biting or picking** - common anxiety symptoms are picking or biting at the nails. If this occurs regularly, the nail's strength decreases, leading to nail splitting most easily. Individuals can split a nail while picking at it in other cases.

- **Excessive exposure to moisture** - being well hydrated is essential for the nail's health. Submerging nails in or constantly exposing them to water will weaken the nails, causing them to become weak and brittle. Additionally, long-term exposure can cause the skin around the nail to soften, where the nail will become brittle, making it easier

to break, bend, or split. People have too much exposure to moisture when they:
- spend a long time in a pool
- do the dishes frequently
- submerge the hands in bathwater

- **Nail polish** - frequent applications can weaken the nails, making them easier to split.

- **Nail psoriasis** - a condition that affects the skin, causing outbreaks of red scaly areas and patches, or plaques. Psoriasis can weaken nails and make them more prone to splitting.

- **Other underlying conditions** - though much less common, several potential conditions can cause nails to split more easily. Some of these conditions include:
  - bacterial, fungal, or yeast infections
  - kidney disease (brown discoloration)
  - liver disease
  - lung disease (yellow nails)
  - skin cancers
  - thyroid disease

- **Trauma or injury** - fingers and fingernails are easy to injure. They could be caught on or in something, pinched under a heavy object, or they can be caught onto anything and cause a rip. Any traumatic event can cause a small or large split. If the damage is severe, it may also affect the nail bed.

Medical Treatment (dermatologist)

With severe nail splits, you may need to see a doctor. Additionally, you should contact your healthcare provider if you notice any of the following symptoms, as they may require medical treatment:

THE HUMAN NAIL - Ailments and Diseases
Symptoms, Causes, and Treatment

- A bluish or purplish color to nail
- A white color arising under nails
- Horizontal ridges on the nails
- Ingrown nails
- Nails that appear distorted
- Painful nails

Other situations in which you might require medical treatment are:

- Infection from fungi, yeast, or bacteria. These infections can require antifungal or antibiotic treatments to help prevent further damage to the nails.

- Psoriasis can damage the nail bed. You will need to take medication to control psoriasis, which can help prevent damage to the nails.

Prevention Of Onychoschizia
To help prevent split nails, you can take certain precautions and make lifestyle adjustments to avoid damage to your nails.

These changes might include:

- Avoid biting and picking around the nails
- Avoiding excessive exposure to water
- Avoid pulling at hangnails
- Avoid the use of harsh nail polish remover
- Giving the nails a break from polishes and gels
- Keep nails clean and healthy
- Maintaining a healthy diet rich in vitamins and minerals (split nails rarely occur due to poor nutrition)
- Moisturizing the nails and cuticles regularly
- Taking biotin supplements
- Wearing adequate protection and using caution when working with the hands

- Wearing gloves when using cleaning chemicals or washing the dishes

Note: preventing split nails usually involves a combination of lifestyle measures.

Paronychia (nail/skin infections)

What Is Paronychia?
Paronychia is an infection of surrounding tissue where the nail meets the skin. Doctors also refer to paronychia as **candidal paronychias** due to a disruption in the barrier between the nail plate and nail fold resulting in infection from the yeast Candida albicans.

Causes Of Paronychia
Paronychia ensues when the skin around the nail is damaged, allowing germs to enter. Bacteria or fungi can cause infections, like Staphylococcus aureus and Streptococcus pyogenes bacteria.

Reasons for skin damage around the nail include:

- Biting or chewing the nails
- Excessive exposure of the hands to moisture, including frequently sucking the finger
- Ingrown nails
- Manicures
- Picking at the nails

Diagnosis Of Paronychia
Paronychia is identified by the type of bacteria or fungi causing the infection. The doctor will take a clipping from the nail or a swab from the affected area and test for bacteria and fungi. Having accomplished this, they can make a diagnosis.

There are two forms of paronychia:

- Acute Paronychia
- Chronic Paronychia

THE HUMAN NAIL - Ailments and Diseases
Symptoms, Causes, and Treatment

Acute Paronychia

Acute paronychia ensues due to infection of the nail fold and the skin at the nail base.

- **Symptoms** - of acute paronychia include:
    - deformation or damage to the nail
    - fever
    - hardening of the nail
    - pain
    - pain in the armpit glands
    - pus from the cuticle
    - reddening and swelling at the nails base
    - separation of the nail from the nailbed

- **Causes** - paronychia occurs when the skin around the nail becomes damaged, allowing germs to enter. Bacteria or fungi can cause infections, such as Staphylococcus aureus and Streptococcus pyogenes bacteria.

    Reasons for skin damage around the nail include:

    - biting or chewing nails
    - excessive exposure of the hands to moisture, including frequently sucking the finger
    - ingrown nails
    - manicures
    - picking at nails

Chronic Paronychia

Repeated exposure to irritants may cause chronic paronychia. Individuals who constantly have wet hands are more likely to have chronic paronychia. Chronic paronychia often begins on one nail and spreads to the others.

- **Symptoms** - of chronic paronychia include:

- a white, yellow, or green pus discharge from the cuticle
- brittle nails
- distorted, ridged nails
- redness and tenderness at the nail base
- yellow or green nails

Treatment for chronic paronychia includes:

- applying topical creams or lotions
- keeping hands clean and dry
- taking antifungal drugs
- use gloves when cleaning or working with chemicals

Treatment for paronychia varies according to the severity and whether it is acute or chronic. Both at-home therapies and medical treatments may help, depending on the diagnosis and severity of the condition.

Medical Treatment Of Paronychia (dermatologist)

When a bacterial infection causes acute paronychia, the doctor may recommend an antibiotic, dicloxacillin, or clindamycin. If a fungal infection causes chronic paronychia, the doctor can prescribe antifungal medication. These topical medications are typically clotrimazole or ketoconazole.

The doctor may also need to drain any pus from the surrounding abscess. They perform a procedure referred to as an incision and drainage method, where they give a local anesthetic and then open a fold large enough to insert gauze to help in draining pus.

Because many household cures lack scientific verification. It is best to consult a medical professional if you think you have paronychia or another type of toe or toenail infection.

THE HUMAN NAIL - Ailments and Diseases
Symptoms, Causes, and Treatment

Stubbed Toe

A stubbed toe is a commonly shared experience. Everyone has felt that sharp pain and throbbing when stubbing a toe.

Symptoms
When you stub your toe, you will typically experience all or some of the following symptoms:

- Bleeding from the nailbed
- Bruising
- Swelling
- Throbbing toe pain
- Trouble comfortably putting on a shoe
- Trouble walking

Specific symptoms warrant a trip to your doctor. See your doctor when:

- A bone is exposed
- Pain that intensifies if you try to move the toe
- The pain makes it difficult to walk
- You are not able to move the toe
- Your foot feels numb
- Your toe becomes unusually pale
- Your toe has abnormal bruising
- Your toe is cold to the touch
- Your toe is noticeably deformed

Medical treatment - depending on the severity of the injury, your doctor might want an X-ray to determine whether you have a broken bone. Your doctor might also immobilize your toe. This is often done by **'buddy taping.'** The doctor will tape the injured toe to the healthy toe next to it.

THE HUMAN NAIL - Ailments and Diseases
Symptoms, Causes, and Treatment

Subungual Hematoma

A subungual hematoma is **bruising that appears underneath the nail.** For example, injuring the nail by stubbing a toe or wearing too-tight shoes can cause subungual hematomas.

Symptoms Of Subungual Hematoma
Someone with a subungual hematoma will see:

- Lifting of the nail
- Pain and tenderness in the nail
- Spots of purple, red, brown, or black on the nail

Causes Of Subungual Hematoma
Subungual hematomas happen when an injury opens blood vessels under the nail, causing blood to collect and become trapped in one spot.

Treatment Of Subungual Hematoma (dermatologist)
A subungual hematoma is treated by:

- Compression of the finger or toe with a bandage
- Elevating the injured digit
- Resting
- Taking pain medication
- Utilizing ice wrapped in a cloth or towel to the nail

If a subungual hematoma is minor and the pain is mild, it will usually resolve without treatment or complications. A subungual hematoma should go away as the nail grows out, which takes 6 to 9 months.

Seek medical attention if the subungual hematoma:

- Is incredibly painful
- Keeps bleeding continuously
- Occurs together with an injury to the nails base

A doctor might X-ray the nail to check for injury to the bone below it. The doctor can also lance the subungual hematoma if that is causing pressure to build on the nail. The doctor will then make a small hole in the nail with a laser or a needle. Afterward, the area can be wrapped with a bandage and may continue to drain for up to 3 days. The procedure should not be attempted at home, as it can cause infections or further injury to the nail bed.

Possible signs of an infection include:

- A sense of heat or throbbing in the finger or toe
- A fever
- Excessive redness around the area of injury
- Fluid or pus that drains from under the nail
- Increased swelling or pain
- Red streaks on the skin

If any of these indications appear, see a doctor right away.

Subungual Hematomas Vs. Melanoma

Though rare, melanoma can appear under a fingernail or toenail. The deadliest form of skin cancer is melanoma.

A tumor might look like a subungual hematoma. Melanoma can cause a dark mark to form under the nail. However, it does not usually cause pain and is not linked to an injury.

Talk with your doctor about any unusual marks or colors on the nail that appear without an injury. Minor subungual hematomas usually heal over time without treatment. Trapped blood will be reabsorbed in time, and the dark mark will disappear. It may take 2 to 3 months for a fingernail and up to 9 months for a toenail. If there is severe damage to the nail bed, the nail may be malformed or cracked when it grows back or fails to regrow. However, this is uncommon and may be prevented by seeing a doctor for treatment when an injury occurs.

Acral lentiginous melanoma - is when a fingernail or toenail has a new or changing dark streak. This dark streak could be melanoma, the most serious type of skin cancer.

THE HUMAN NAIL - Ailments and Diseases
Symptoms, Causes, and Treatment

Turf Toe

If you engage in physical activities on hard, slick surfaces, you may someday find yourself with a turf toe. To help prevent this from occurring:

- Do not wear shoes with flexible soles that have a lot of give.

- Do not work out barefoot.

- Footwear with cleats could make you more prone to injury since they grab the ground and can cause your toe to overextend.

- Wear shoes with stiff soles that keep your toes in a neutral position.

What Is Turf Toe
It is **an injury to the big toe's main joint.** The joint is called the metatarsophalangeal joint (MTP). A turf toe injury could also stretch or tear the ligaments and tendons surrounding the MTP joint. This particular part of the foot is the plantar complex.

Turf toe tends to occur on firm, slick surfaces that do not give, such as the turf that football is performed on, hence its name.

Grades Of Turf Toe
There are three grades of turf toe:

- **Grade 1 turf toe** - the ligaments surrounding the MTP joint are stretched, but they do not tear. Tenderness and slight swelling may occur. Mild pain may be felt.

- **Grade 2 turf toe** - partial tearing occurs, causing swelling, bruising, pain, and decreased movement in the toe.

- **Grade 3 turf toe** - the plantar complex tears severely, causing the toe's inability to move, bruising, swelling, and pain.

Symptoms Of Turf Toe

Turf toe causes pain, swelling, and bruising, making it hard to stand or bear weight on your foot. In some instances, the turf toe may also cause dislocation of the big toe, which may require surgery.

Causes of Turf Toe

A turf toe injury occurs when the big toe hyperextends toward the foot, bending up and inward too far.

Treatment For Turf Toe

Turf toe taping is one of several conservative treatments that support the healing of this injury. If done correctly, toe taping restricts flexion or the ability of the big toe to bend. This provides:

- Pain relief
- Protection of the toe and foot
- Stabilization

Does Taping Help Turf Toe?

Most likely, but it depends on the severity of the injury. However, a literature review on turf toe injury determined that all three severity levels, or grades, benefit from conservative treatments, including taping and the **R.I.C.E.** (rest, ice, compression, elevation) method. Wearing stiff-soled shoes or orthotics is also recommended.

Note: call your doctor if your pain is severe or does not abate with conservative treatment within 12 hours. You might have broken a bone or experienced an injury severe enough to require more aggressive treatment.

Turf Toe Healing Time

The more severe your turf toe injury, the longer it will take for complete healing to occur.

- Grade 1 injuries may resolve partially or entirely within one week

- Grade 2 injuries may take around two weeks to resolve

- Grade 3 injuries may require anywhere from 2 to 6 months before healing is complete. Occasionally, a Grade 3 turf toe injury may require surgery

THE HUMAN NAIL - Ailments and Diseases
Symptoms, Causes, and Treatment

Yellow Toenails

Healthy nails are usually clear in color and do not have issues like cracks, indentations, ridges, or abnormal shapes.

Causes Of Yellow Toenails
If your toenails turn yellow, it could result from something a little less serious, like aging or nail polish. Or might be due to a more severe issue, like an infection. Other factors for yellow toenails are:

- **Aging** - can be a natural cause of yellow toenails and fingernails. As people grow older, their nail color, thickness, and shape change. Aging individuals often have a more yellow tint to their nails.

- **Medical Condition** - having yellow toenails is not dangerous by itself. However, if the cause of yellow toenails is an underlying medical condition, this is a sign that there is something wrong. For example, yellow toenails could be caused by an infection, fungus, or medical disorder.

- **Infection** - a most common cause of yellow toenails is an infection by a fungus that attacks the nails. It is called **onychomycosis,** and it takes place more in adults than children. It can make the nail turn yellow, yellow spots, white patches, or even black patches.
  - **Fungus** - a fungal infection caused by dermatophytes, eats keratin to grow. Keratin is found in both the skin and nails. According to **American Family Physician, onychomycosis** happens in about 10 percent of the adult population, with the risk of getting it escalating with age. Nearly half of people over the age of 70 get a fungal infection.

Yellow nail syndrome - in rare cases, yellow toenails can signify a yellow nail syndrome disorder **(YNS).** Doctors do not know what causes YNS, but people who have it have **yellow, curved, thickened nails that grow slowly and other symptoms like respiratory problems.** Their nails may also have **ridges or indentations and turn black or green.**

Sometimes the nail will lack a cuticle and may even pull away from the nail bed. It may be the result of:

- Internal malignancies
- Lymphedema, swelling of the hands
- Pleural effusions, fluid build-up between lungs and chest cavity
- Respiratory illnesses like chronic bronchitis or sinusitis
- Rheumatoid arthritis

Treatment For Yellow Toenails (podiatrist or dermatologist)
In most cases, yellow toenails are treatable. Some medications and home remedies might help cure yellow toenails or help lighten the yellow color. Whatever treatment your doctor recommends will depend on what is causing the yellow nails.

For example, if a fungal infection is causing your yellow toenails, you will require antifungal medicines to treat it. The most popular prescription antifungal medication is ciclopirox 8 percent solution, which is put on the nails similar to nail polish.

Other medications that can help cure yellow toenails include applying vitamin E, zinc, and a topical corticosteroid with Vitamin D-3. Using antibiotics is especially helpful if there is an infection present somewhere in the body, like pneumonia.

You may be unable to prevent yellow toenails from ever happening again. However, your best bet is to practice proper nail care and regularly inspect and monitor your nails for signs of any issues, especially if you have poor circulation or are prone to

THE HUMAN NAIL - Ailments and Diseases
Symptoms, Causes, and Treatment

nail disorders. Be sure to:

- Air out your shoes regularly after sports or other activities to ensure that they are not wet while you wear them

- Always wear clean socks

- Always wear properly fitting shoes. Have your shoes checked by a professional if you are unsure of the correct size. Feet can change shape and size with weight gain, loss, or pregnancy

- Be careful when selecting a salon for a pedicure and check to make sure they change the water and sanitize stations between customers

- Cut toenails in a straight line with clean nail clippers

- Keep nails clean and dry

Consult your doctor if your nails also have any of the following conditions:

- Any bleeding
- Change in shape or thickness
- Discharge
- Pain
- Swelling

****# Section 4
HOME REMEDIES****

Ingrown Toenail

The most considerable risk associated with an ingrown toenail is infection. If caught early, an ingrown may be treated at home.

Treatment

You can do several things at home to help alleviate the pain and discomfort caused by an ingrown toenail.

- Apply a topical antibiotic, like polymyxin and neomycin (both present in Neosporin) or a steroid cream, to prevent infection

- Pushing the skin further from the toenail edge with a cotton ball soaked in olive oil

- Soak the feet in warm water for 15 to 20 minutes three to four times per day. Always keep your shoes and feet dry.

- Use over-the-counter medicines, like acetaminophen (Tylenol), for the pain

Try home remedies for a few days to a few weeks. See your doctor if the pain worsens or you find it difficult to walk or perform other activities because of the toenail. If the toenail does not respond to the treatment or an infection occurs, see your doctor immediately.

For additional information, see **'Ingrown Toenails.'**

Nail Dystrophy

If one has brittle, peeling, or split nails, using moisturizers is beneficial for protecting the keratin that holds the nails altogether. After addressing trauma, infections, and diseases that may cause nail dystrophy, the best solution is to focus on adequately moisturizing the nails each day.

Treatment

- **Brittle nails** - can be treated with vitamin supplements: Biotin, zinc, and iron, which are recognized to improve nail strength. Sufferers might also try moisturizers, fortified nail polish, and a nail-protecting regimen to avoid harsh soaps.

- **Peeling nails** - are usually a symptom of physical or chemical stress. Nutrient deficiencies and overexposure to water can bring about peeling nails. This problem may even be something as simple as cold, dry weather. Peeling nails can be prevented or treated by being aware of lifestyle and the environmental factors that affect hands. Employing glycerin, petrolatum, and mineral oil moisturizers can help.

For additional information, see **'Nail Dystrophy.'**

Nail Fungus (onychomycosis)

Toenail fungus is a frequent fungal infection of the toenails. The most visible symptom is a white, brown, or yellow discoloration of one or more toenails. The nail may also crumble and become jagged at the edge and spread to other toenails. It can also expand to the surrounding skin. The fungus can spread and cause the nails to thicken or crack.

Popular At-Home Treatments
The following are popular at-home treatments:

- **Topical antifungals** - several over-the-counter (OTC) treatments are available to treat nail fungus in liquids, solutions, and creams. These products are applied directly to the nail and surrounding skin to treat cases of nail fungus infection. Common topical antifungals include clotrimazole and terbinafine. *Note: OTC products such as terbinafine cream may provide relief in conjunction with regular debridement and consistent use over four to six months.*

- **Listerine mouthwash** - contains menthol, thymol, and eucalyptus, which have antibacterial and antifungal properties. This may be why it is a popular folk remedy for toenail fungus. The treatment's support recommends soaking the affected foot in a basin of amber-colored Listerine for 30 minutes daily.

- **Oregano oil** - contains thymol which has antifungal and antibacterial properties. To treat, apply oregano oil to the affected nail twice daily with a cotton swab.

- **Olive leaf extract** – oleuropein, an active substance in olive leaf extract, is thought to have antifungal, antimicrobial, and immune-boosting abilities. Ingesting one to three olive leaf capsules with meals twice daily is most effective. It is also recommended that you drink plenty of water throughout this treatment.

- **Ozonized oils** - are oils like olive oil and sunflower oil injected with ozone gas. This exposure in low concentrations for a short duration can inactivate many organisms such as fungi, yeast, and bacteria. For treating the toenail fungus with ozonized oil, work the oil into the affected toenail twice a day.

- **Snakeroot extract (Ageratina pichinchensis)** - is an antifungal made from plants in the sunflower family. Apply snakeroot extract to affected areas every third day during the first month, twice a week for the second month, and weekly for the third month.

- **Tea tree oil (melaleuca)** - is an essential oil with antifungal and antiseptic abilities. Brush the tea tree oil directly onto the affected nail twice daily with a cotton swab.

- **Vicks VapoRub** - is a popular, topical ointment designed for cough suppression. Its active ingredients (camphor and eucalyptus oil) can help to treat toenail fungus. Apply small amounts of Vicks VapoRub to the affected area at least once a day.

Adjust Your Diet

The connection between diet and health is clear. Healthy foods give your body a better chance to fight off ailments like toenail fungus. Provide your body with the nutrients it needs and eat:

- A diet rich in essential fatty acids
- Enough iron to prevent brittle nails
- Enough protein to support nail regrowth
- Foods that are rich in calcium and vitamin D, such as low-fat dairy products
- Probiotic-rich yogurt

When To See A Doctor
Generally, toenail fungus is considered a cosmetic problem. Still, it may cause severe complications for some people. It is advisable not to use home remedies for toenail fungus when you have diabetes or a weakened immune system. Call your doctor for the appropriate course of action.

For additional information, see **'Onychomycosis.'**

THE HUMAN NAIL - Ailments and Diseases
Symptoms, Causes, and Treatment

Nail Splitting, Brittle, Soft (onychoschizia)

Treatment

Most treatment options for split nails are home remedies. In most cases, nails will split because of repeated drying and wetting, leading to dryness and brittleness. The causes can be even worse in the winter with dry heat or areas with low humidity. The safest solution is to apply lotions with lanolin or alpha-hydroxy acids after soaking nails in water for five minutes or more.

Home remedies usually involve repairing the nail in place and improving its appearance until the break grows out. For instance:

- **Try a gel and silk wrap** - this method involves using a nail-sized section of silk wrap, placing it against the broken nail, and applying a gel coat. Once set, you can choose to buff the nail and apply polish.

- **Try glue** - this method involves applying a minimal amount of adhesive to the detached nail and then using gentle pressure to push the nail back together. After the bond has been set, you can paint the nail if you wish to hide the break.

- **Use a fake nail** - this method involves removing the piece that is splitting off or leaving it in place. Then, apply a fake nail to just the broken nail.

- **Use a teabag** - For this method to work, cut a nail-sized portion of a teabag from an ordinary tea bag. Then, use a brush with glue to adhere the tea bag in place. Once the glue sets, you can buff the nail and paint over it.

For additional information, see **'Onychoschizia.'**

THE HUMAN NAIL - Ailments and Diseases
Symptoms, Causes, and Treatment

Paronychia (nail/skin infections)

At-Home Treatment - a person can treat acute paronychia by:

- Applying antibiotic creams (OTC)
- Using soaks

An individual with mild paronychia can soak the infected finger or toe in warm water several times a day. If symptoms do not improve, they then should seek medical treatment.

For additional information, see **'Paronychia.'**

Stubbed Toe

After stubbing a toe, follow the **RICE** method for injury treatment:

- **Rest** - stop using your feet, lie down, and let your body recover.

- **Ice** - use ice to numb the pain and reduce swelling. Wrap the ice in a towel to not touch the skin directly.

- **Compression** - wrap your toe, or the entire end of your foot and toes, with an elastic bandage to support and keep swelling under control.

- **Elevation** - keep your foot raised above the level of your heart to reduce discomfort and swelling.

If pain relief is required, consider an over-the-counter pain reliever, such as:

- Acetaminophen
- Aspirin
- Ibuprofen
- Naproxen

For additional information, see **'Stubbed Toe.'**

Section 5
NAIL POLISH and TOXIC CHEMICALS

Being Trendy

Putting textured or layered ornamentation on your fingernails creates a breeding ground for bacteria, dirt, and food. Allowing this matter to attach to the fingernails for prolonged periods is simply unsanitary!

Thick items can shield the fingernails from moisture, which is one of the worst things you can do if you are trying to promote proper nail health. The fingernails need moisture to hydrate, grow, and repair themselves properly. Depriving those fingernails of humidity and oxygen could lead to brittle, peeling nails.

Some people who opt for trendy fingernails will frequently change their fingernail designs and colors, which exposes the nails to harmful chemicals. Increased exposure to these toxic chemicals to have a new look can put one on the fast track to nail dystrophy.

The future of your fingernails depends on you dealing with this emerging fad responsibly.

Nail Polish and Toxins

Few luxuries seem more straightforward or more harmless than a manicure or pedicure. Still, if you are not careful about your brands, your nail polish may expose you to dangerous toxins. Chemicals found in nail polish are harmful to everyone who uses them, especially those repeatedly exposed (manicurists, beauticians, or people that frequently have their nails done). These toxins should also be avoided by pregnant or nursing women and children who have not yet passed puberty. Keeping yourself and those around you safe involves selecting polishes and avoiding the **five major chemicals: dibutyl phthalate, toluene, formaldehyde, formaldehyde resin, and camphor.**

DBP (Dibutyl Phthalate)
Dibutyl phthalate (DBP), a phthalate family of chemicals, is used in nail polish to minimize chipping. Phthalates are classified as endocrine disruptors and simulate the hormone estrogen in the body. Phthalates are proven to impair the hormonal development of male fetuses, cause organ damage, and may even initiate early-onset menopause.

Although there are no human studies, animal studies show comparable results to human phthalate studies. It includes reduced fertility, hormonal disruption, bioaccumulation, and liver damage.

The European Union banned DBP in both cosmetic and personal care products, and the Australian government classified DBP as a risk to the human reproductive system. In the United States, California ranks it as a reproductive and hormonal toxicant, but the federal government does not.

Toluene

This nail polish ingredient creates a slick application as well as its finish. Toluene has a sweet, pungent smell and is found in most conventional nail polish removers. The fumes of this ingredient are highly toxic.

Studies show that exposure to toluene can cause neurological damage, decreased brain function, impaired breathing, hearing loss, and nausea. When inhaled frequently by pregnant women, it may harm fetal development. Animal studies have shown that toluene is linked to reproductive impairment, immune system toxicity, and blood cancers like malignant lymphoma.

The European Union has restricted toluene in personal care products, including nail polish, and advises that pregnant women and children must not be exposed to the vapors. In California, toluene is on the state's Proposition 65 list of harmful chemicals to fetal development.

Formaldehyde

It is used in nail polishes to harden and strengthen them and serve as a preservative protecting against bacterial growth. The body naturally produces formaldehyde in minimal amounts, similar to the concentration found in some vaccines. Formaldehyde at this low level is not dangerous.

Exposure to large amounts of formaldehyde in the air or on the skin can cause cancer of the throat, nose, and blood. Nail salon workers and their children are particularly at risk for chronic health issues caused by formaldehyde, including asthma, convulsions, nausea, and miscarriages. Repeated exposure may cause a build-up of fluid in the lungs and cause abnormal fetal development in pregnant women.

The European Union only allows limited use of formaldehyde in personal care products, while Japan and Sweden have banned it altogether.

Formaldehyde Resin

Formaldehyde resin, a by-product of formaldehyde, makes its way into many nail polish formulas that include formaldehyde. The resin has been the subject of fewer human tests than the other chemicals mentioned in this Section. However, studies show that it can cause severe skin irritation and allergic reactions, skin depigmentation, and loss of nerve sensation.

Camphor

It is an ingredient used to give conventional nail polishes a glossy, shiny appearance. Camphor is less-toxic than the first three items and is used in cold remedies such as vapor rubs and nasal sprays.

The safety of camphor is now being called into question. When applied topically, it can trigger severe skin irritation, cause allergic reactions, and inhaling its fumes can cause nausea, dizziness, and headaches. Observational studies link camphor exposure to organ damage, like liver dysfunction.

Camphor in personal care products in the U.S. is limited to a concentration of 11% and is being phased out in markets within the European Union.

THE HUMAN NAIL - Ailments and Diseases
Symptoms, Causes, and Treatment

APPENDIX A

THE HUMAN NAIL - Ailments and Diseases
Symptoms, Causes, and Treatment

Must-Know Words and Phrases

Alpha-Keratin - is a fibrous protein found as a primary material in vertebrates. It is a structural component of body parts such as hair, epidermal skin, nails, claws, and horns of mammals.

Biotin - is an essential part of enzymes in the body that break down substances like fats, carbohydrates, and others. A deficiency is identified by its symptoms, including thin hair and a red scaly rash around the eyes, nose, and mouth. Biotin is also used for biotin deficiency, hair loss, brittle nails, and other conditions. No scientific evidence supports these uses.

Enzyme - is a substance produced by a living organism that acts as a catalyst to bring about a specific biochemical reaction.

Hyponychium - the cells in it produce keratin, which builds up in layers and develops into the nail plates we have on the toes and fingers

Keratinizing - the formation of or conversion into keratin. It occurs in the outer layers of the skin but is prominent when the skin is exposed to constant localized pressure. Corns and callosities are areas of keratinization.

Nail dystrophy - refers to poor nail formation, usually resulting from trauma or infection. The nail becomes discolored when caused by trauma due to blood pooling underneath the nail. Over time, the nail will break away from the nail bed until it detaches completely.

Onychomycosis - is a nondermatophytic infection of the nail but is now used as a general term to denote any fungal nail infection.

Onychophagia - nail-biting can include biting the nail, the cuticle, and tissue around the nail. Most nail biters do not develop long-term damage, but it can happen.

THE HUMAN NAIL - Ailments and Diseases
Symptoms, Causes, and Treatment

Psoriasis - is a skin disorder that causes skin cells to multiply up to 10 times faster than usual. The skin builds up into bumpy red patches covered with white scales. Psoriasis is not spread from one person to another.

So That You Know

Have you ever wondered about the terminologies used to indicate a physician and doctor? The following is a brief explanation:

The word **Physician** is a word used commonly for a health care provider. The individual called physician is a healthcare provider trained to diagnose and then **prescribe medications to treat the symptoms of various illnesses.** Whenever symptoms signal something is wrong with an individual's body, they get an appointment with their physician to ensure that they receive the proper diagnosis and treatment.

If the symptoms are such that a physician feels a specialist must see the patient, they will refer their patient to a specialist in their ailment or condition.

All physicians receive comprehensive training, which helps them choose the appropriate **drugs and medication** necessary to **treat and prevent diseases.** They can deal with medical issues and have the skills to make clinical decisions. While one must earn a medical doctorate to be considered a physician, they may select and focus on a specialty, such as Cardiology, Dermatology, Neurology, and more.

Primary Care Doctors - may be family medicine practitioners, pediatricians, or internal medicine doctors. The primary care doctor is always your first line of defense for medical care and the first doctor you should visit.

Internal Medicine Doctor - also called an internist, an internal medicine doctor specializes in adults' care. An internal medicine doctor could be your primary care provider. They have the knowledge, training, and experience in diagnosing and treating both simple and complex injuries and diseases most often affecting adults. They emphasize the prevention of diseases and chronic disease management that adults are most likely to develop.

In the medical field, a **Medical Doctor** is any physician who restores a person's health by practicing medicine. Doctors guide patients, determine a patient's illness, implement treatment plans, and more.

Differences between the **Physician** and **Medical Doctor** are:

- A physician works in conjunction with a doctor. A doctor works independently

- Physicians use medication and drugs to cure patients. Doctors use full-scale medical procedures and surgeries to treat patients.

- Physicians complete eight years of medical school, but doctors with specialization have gone through 11-13 years of studying.

Specialist To Visit For Conditions In This Book

A dermatologist is a doctor that diagnoses and treats conditions that affect the hair, skin, and nails. In addition to the skin, dermatology also includes conditions that affect your nails, such as:

- Discoloration
- Nail separation
- Spots

THE HUMAN NAIL - Ailments and Diseases
Symptoms, Causes, and Treatment

A **podiatrist** is a healthcare specialist that diagnoses and treats medical conditions and injuries that primarily involve the feet. Podiatrists diagnose and treat a variety of ailments, including:

- Causes of heel pain, such as plantar fasciitis

- Diabetic foot disorders, like infections, chronic ulcers, nerve damage, or neuropathy

- Foot injuries, such as fractured, broken bones, as well as sprains and strains

- Foot pain and swelling due to arthritis, rheumatoid arthritis, or gout

- Nail conditions, including ingrown nails, claw toe, and nail infections

- Skin conditions, such as warts, bunions, corns, plantar dermatosis, and athlete's foot

- Structural foot defects, including hammertoe, flat feet, and high arches

THE HUMAN NAIL - Ailments and Diseases
Symptoms, Causes, and Treatment

AFTERWORD

Thank you for reading,

THE HUMAN NAIL
Ailments and Diseases
Symptoms, Causes, and Treatment

We hope you enjoyed this
Life Knowledge Media USA Publication

Thank you again, valued reader,
and we hope to meet you again on another book.

ABOUT THE AUTHOR

Pierre Mouchette is the Founder and CEO of Real Property Experts LLC. He is a graduate of New York University, with a Master's in Business Administration, a Certificate in Real Estate Law - Fairfield University - CT, a Graduate of the Realtors Institute - CT, and held licensing as a Real Estate Broker, and a Mortgage Broker.

Pierre is currently authoring Books, Booklets, How-to-Articles, and Guides in retirement. Pierre has an extensive background in real estate investment, business management, and sales, supplemented by decades of hands-on experience in building systems engineering, development, evaluation, and various analytical engineering studies.

Pierre launched Real Property Experts in 2013 to simplify real estate investing by connecting investors through innovative technology using background knowledge and experience. In 2018, Pierre created THE SYNCHRONICITY INVESTOR, a real estate website to facilitate world-class solutions for real estate investors and investment businesses.

During the winter of 2021, Pierre created Enviro | Life Publications to bring Environmental and Life Knowledge to a growing TSI audience. Exploring the Internet and using all sources available, this entity will bring to our audience, through its Research, Information that is Transparent and easy to understand, thereby making them more Knowledgeable.

Life-Health Media USA

- presents -

An Enviro | Life Knowledge Publications

LIFE HEALTH

HEALTH and DISEASES

MENIER'S DISEASE – What Is Meniere's, Symptoms, Treatment, and Lifestyle

OVERACTIVE BLADDER – Symptoms, Treatments, and Lifestyle Remedies

TREMORS - What Is Hand Tremor, Signs, Symptoms, and Treatment

THE HUMAN NAIL - Ailments and Diseases Symptoms, Causes, and Treatment

www.ingramcontent.com/pod-product-compliance
Lightning Source LLC
Chambersburg PA
CBHW050012230526
45465CB00003BB/1389